Running
made easy

Susie Whalley & Lisa Jackson

in association with

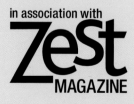

ZeSt
MAGAZINE

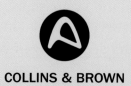

COLLINS & BROWN

"Thanks so much for getting me outside and running. Since buying your book I've gone from half-heartedly doing 20 minutes on the treadmill to doing two half-marathons! Carole Parkhouse, York

'*Running Made Easy* is a FANTASTIC, FABULOUS, EASY, COMPELLING, MOTIVATIONAL, COLOURFUL and ENJOYABLE book. I'm an exercise professional so I've read countless fitness books, but none is as friendly, accurate and worth while as yours. Take it from a professional, you will buy this book, use it, write all over it, buy another one, give it to a friend, pick it up again and reread it, then buy another one for another friend!' Anna Snook, director of Degrees Of Fitness, Berkshire/Buckinghamshire

'I love the format: it's modern, exciting and filled with practical advice and information that's fun to read and, most importantly, easy to apply.' Bridget Robinson, Canada

'Fabulous book with all the information you need to get started and keep going. All you're expected to be able to do is a 60-second jog, which is doable for everyone, really.' Amazon review by relikaarras

'You have achieved the impossible – getting me to stick to an exercise programme week after week after week! I have enjoyed every second, even when it was tough.' Kate Banks, Oxford

'A brilliant book for anyone about to start running, it is so inspirational with lots of success stories from all kinds of people who now love running.'
Sharon Freedman, Glasgow

'Buy it and smile as you run!' Amazon review by brazen_67

'The training programme was broken into incredibly simple and absolutely achievable steps, even by a first-time, apprehensive runner like me! It's kept me running confidently – and best of all, I'm enjoying it.'
Angie Govender, South Africa

'A big thank you for the continued common sense, inspiration from all your contributors and the encouragement your book has offered.'
Alysoun Sturt-Scobie, France

'I've gone from couch potato to total running enthusiast and had a total life change in just eight weeks.'
Katy Ryan, Northamptonshire

'Thanks so much for a great book. Your writing style is accessible and funny, the graphics are funky, and your motivational stories are priceless.' Gabrielle Watt, Australia

'I couldn't put it down – but when I did, I got my trainers out and went for a run!
Amazon review by laineylou95

This edition pubished in 2008
by Collins and Brown
10 Southcombe Street
London W14 0RA

An imprint of Anova Books
First published in Great Britain in 2004

Distributed in the United States and Canada by
Sterling Publishing Co, 387 Park Avenue South,
New York, NY 10016, USA

Zest is the registered trademark of The National
Magazine Company Ltd.

The authors have made every reasonable effort to
contact all copyright holders. Any errors that may
have occurred are inadvertent and anyone who for
any reason has not been contacted is invited to
write to the publishers so that a full acknowledgement
may be made in subsequent editions of this work.

British Library Cataloguing in Publication Data.
A catalogue record for this title is available from
the British Library.

ISBN 9781843404347

Picture credits:
Illustrator Paul Luke
Stylists Marianne de Vries, Kelly Moseley
Still-life photographers Louisa Parry, Derek Lomas
Cover photographer Neil Cooper
Photograph of Susie by Karen Hatch
Photograph of Lisa by Merle Moustafa

Repro by Spectrum Colour Ltd, UK
Printed in Times Offset (M) Sdn. Bhd, Malaysia

The exercise programmes in this book are
intended for people in good health – if you
have a medical condition or are pregnant,
or have any other health concerns, consult
your GP before starting out.

LISA JACKSON is a journalist and clinical
hypnotherapist. An extremely reluctant
convert to running, she's now an ardent
evangelist and has run 12 marathons in
fancy dress: London (twice), Rome, Berlin,
Paris (twice), New York (twice, the first time
with her sister and marathon-virgin mum,
aged 63!), Stockholm, Edinburgh, Medoc
and Abingdon. Born in South Africa, she
lives in London with her husband Graham.

LISA'S THANKS

This book is dedicated to my beloved
mother, Leone Jackson, who was tragically
killed, aged 68, while training to run the
Medoc Marathon with our family. My Mom
encouraged all of us to run and continues to
inspire us. She had more enthusiasm in her
little finger than all of us put together, and
her love of life – and running – will always
be with us. I'd also like to thank my
husband Graham, my family, Aunt Rosie,
Bridget and Kent Robinson, Ivy
Shakespeare, Sarah Owen and Emma
Simpson. And finally thanks to the dozens
of you for writing to share your amazing
stories with us.

SUSIE WHALLEY is a journalist working in
women's magazines. Having rediscovered
running in her mid-twenties after a long
lapse, she has now run five London
Marathons and one New York City Marathon.
She lives in London with her husband Adam.

SUSIE'S THANKS

Thanks to my dad for inspiring me to start
running and encouraging me all the way.
He's a great runner (3:20, Robin Hood
Marathon, Nottingham, 1985) and a great
role model – I only hope I'm as fit as him
when I'm 65! Thanks also to my husband
Adam, the ultimate unwilling runner, who
took a leap of faith by running his (one and
only!) marathon with me, and who
supported me through writing this book.
Thanks also to all of you fabulous readers
who've contacted us. To know we've helped
you out makes it all feel so worth while.

contents

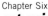

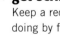

○ ○ ○ We've written our book *Running Made Easy* because we're bursting to tell you about the joys of running and the in-love-with-life way it can make you feel. Turn the page to find out how we got hooked – and how we can help you do the same…

get to know us

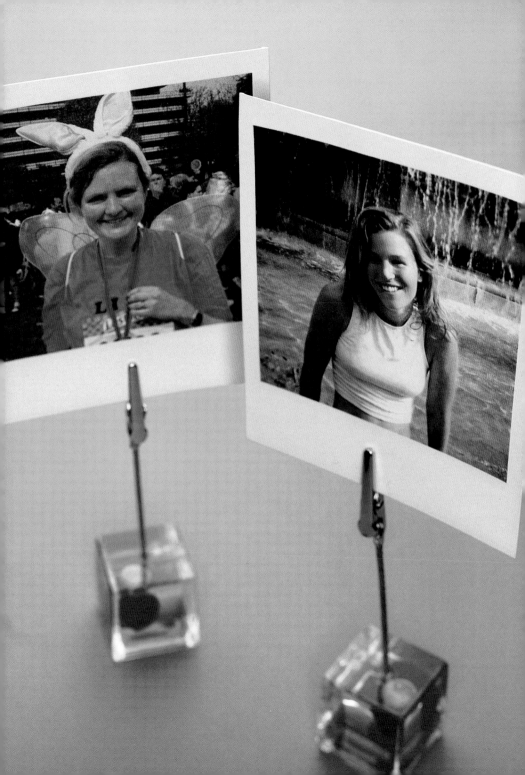

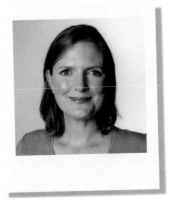

Lisa Jackson, 40, journalist and clinical hypnotherapist

Running pace Think of the slowest runner you know – then think twice as slow!

Running CV I'm a late-onset runner. For 31 years I was a fully paid-up member of The Couch Potato Society. Exercise? No one can say they loathed, hated and detested it more than me.

Then, in June 1998, I was blown away by the electrifying atmosphere of a 5K (3-mile) race that I'd been cajoled into doing. I was surprised by just how much of a kick I got from the crowds and the camaraderie. Soon afterwards, I threw caution to the wind and entered the Great North Run, the world's biggest half-marathon.

Again I was bowled over by the thrill of having dared to challenge myself to run 21km (13.1 miles) and the spectacle of 30,000 people surging along the road ahead of me. Six months later, I completed the Flora London Marathon and had one of the most memorable days of my life. From then on, I was well and truly hooked.

Eleven other marathons, all run in fancy dress, followed, including one in New York in which I was one of the guides for the disabled runner Nkele Mosiane, whom I'd interviewed for this book (read her story on page 193).

What I wish I'd known about running before I started I wish I'd known about the ecstasy of running – the feeling of flushed wellbeing I get after a training run I begged myself not to have to do, but did anyway; the incomparable feeling of crossing the finish line in a race, having used up every last ounce of willpower to get there. I wish I'd known about the friends I'd make, both the people I'd end up running with regularly and those whom I met, for a few brief moments during a race. If I had known, I'd have started running at 21 not 31.

How writing *Running Made Easy* has changed my life Before I wrote this book, I had no idea how many people out there felt exactly the way I did about running – that it wasn't for types like us who believed we just weren't cut out for it. So when the letters and emails started to flood in from readers who said our book had transformed their lives, given them self-confidence, saved their marriage, helped them recover from injury and generally made them fall in love with life again, I was delighted, moved and touched. The book's ability to help readers take control of their lives inspired me to train as a clinical hypnotherapist, which hopefully means I can continue helping others change their lives for good.

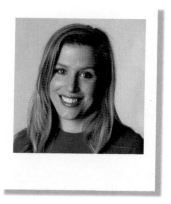

Susie Whalley, 34, journalist

Running pace Fairly sprightly – especially if there are other runners to chase! – but I also like a nice lazy Sunday plod.

Running CV My earliest memories of running are of trotting off down country lanes with my dad to fetch the day's baguette on family holidays in France. I wasn't sure why, but even aged eight, with little legs that could barely keep up, I was desperate to follow in his footsteps and become a runner. At school I loved sports days, and every April I'd watch the Flora London Marathon with tears in my eyes, dreaming of taking part.

My ambitions were shelved at university (too much time at the bar!), so when I decided to start training for the marathon aged 25, it felt pretty tough. But I did it, loved it, and amazingly it's now ten years down the line and I've run a total of six marathons and heaps of other races since. Being a runner has become a really big part of who I am and I wouldn't change that for the world.

Proudest moment Rounding the corner to run up The Mall towards the finish line of my first London Marathon, hand in hand with my great friend Louise. With the crowd cheering us on, and the finish line in sight, knowing we were going to make it, was just the most fantastic feeling in the world. And also writing *Running Made Easy*. We never quite knew what people would think of it, but now it's sold more than 30,000 copies and we've had so many lovely, inspiring and humbling letters from readers telling us how the book helped them.

Most embarrassing moment Hmm, quite a few. Running on the treadmill at the gym and the guy next to me telling me I had my shorts on inside out. Sprinting for the finish line in a race only to be told I'd gone the wrong way and having to turn round and retrace my steps in front of hundreds of people. Almost running into a deer while jogging in the park without my contact lenses in. I could go on...

What running has taught me To love, respect and listen to my body and the amazing way it can make me feel. There's nothing more wonderful than running by the Thames in the early morning, feeling the blood racing through my veins, my heart hammering in my chest and the sweat pouring down my back. Even if it sometimes hurts, it shows me that I'm fit, healthy, and zinging with energy, capable of doing so much more than just sitting at a desk from nine to five. It's also taught me that anything is possible – if you want it badly enough.

Wondering if running is really for you, or why you're more likely to stick to our programme than any other you've already tried? We're here to answer all your questions, banish all your doubts, and set you on the road to runaway success...

1
get ready

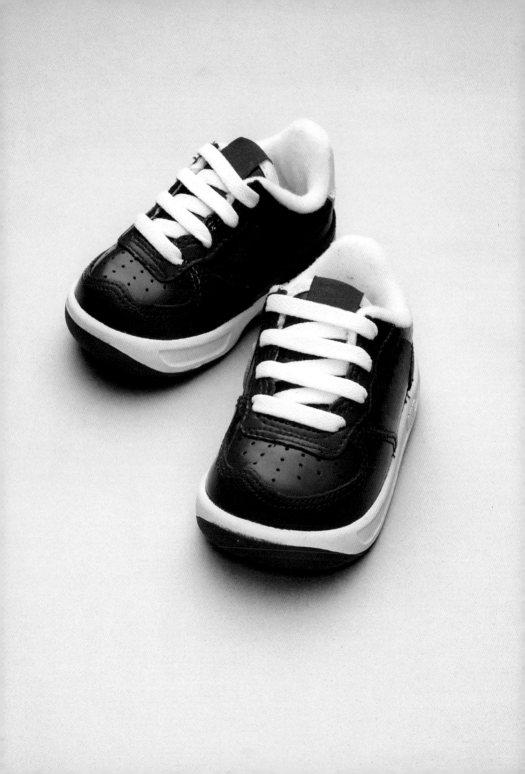

Yes, we do mean just 60 seconds. If so, you've got what it takes to do something that has the power to shape up your whole life and totally transform you, from your buttocks to your brain cells and beyond. An activity that will make you feel passionate, alive, energised, joyful and confident in a way that no box of chocolates or shopping spree ever could. That can turn you into a hero for a day, and get thousands of people chanting your name. It's something that you've known how to do since childhood, but have probably neglected to do since you grew up. Something that's blindingly obvious, easy to fit into your day – and free. Quite simply, it's running.

But will it work for me?

Of course, if you give it a chance. The best thing about running is that it can give you whatever you need – whether that's a better body, quiet time to think, or something more radical like the confidence to make life-changing decisions or tackle an 'I didn't think I had it in me' challenge. But in order for running to work for you, you need to approach it in the right way. Try to run too far, too fast (as you may have done in the past) and you'll find yourself doubled over with exhaustion, giving up before you even get to the good bits. But do it right and it's actually amazingly easy – providing you know where to start. And that's where Running Made Easy comes in. We've developed something called The 60-Second-Secret Plan, which we believe is the very best way

to ease you painlessly into running. If you've barely run a step in your life – or even if you've been running half-heartedly for years – The 60-Second-Secret Plan will take you back to basics and help you build a solid fitness foundation that will enable you to achieve all your goals. Follow this plan and you'll fall in love with running. For life. Guaranteed! It's all about starting small but aiming big. About learning to combine walking with 60-second bursts of running (as fast or slow as you like) and building up from there. It'll take you wherever you want to go – from minute to mile to marathon.

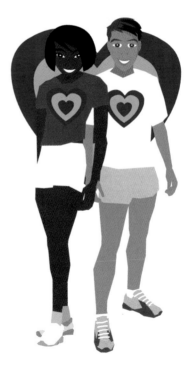

Why run?

Apart from making you look and feel fantastic, running can massively improve your health, something most of us in the Western world really need to do. A worrying 79% of adults in England don't get enough exercise, and we're suffering from a host of health problems related to this lack of physical activity. The good news is that running can help stop many of them in their tracks. Here's the evidence to prove it:

216,000 deaths a year in the UK are caused by cardiovascular disease (mainly heart disease and stroke). That's around four out of every ten deaths. *(British Heart Foundation.)*

50% is how much you can reduce your risk of heart disease if you're physically active. *(British Heart Foundation.)*

63% is how much you can reduce your risk of stroke if you run regularly for 20–40 minutes, three to five times a week. *(Medicine And Science In Sports And Exercise Journal.)*

1.6 billion adults worldwide are overweight and at least 400 million are obese. *(World Health Organization.)*

100% is how sure we are that you'll lose weight if you exercise regularly and reduce your calorie intake.

31% is how much higher your risk of developing breast cancer is, if you are a woman who is post-menopausal and obese. *(European Prospective Investigation of Cancer.)*

30% is how much you can reduce your risk of breast cancer if you exercise on a regular basis. *(University of Bristol research.)*

12,000 people a year in the UK might avoid getting cancer if they maintained a healthy body weight. *(International Journal of Cancer.)*

246 million people worldwide have diabetes, with up to 95% of them suffering from type-2 diabetes, which is often associated with being overweight. *(International Diabetes Federation.)*

Up to 80% of type-2 diabetes is preventable by adopting a healthy diet and increasing physical activity. *(International Diabetes Federation.)*

58% is how much participants in a study reduced their risk of getting type-2 diabetes by, by exercising, on average, for 30 minutes per day. *(Joslin Diabetes Center.)*

30–40 minutes of weight-bearing exercise (such as running) three to four times a week can help to prevent osteoporosis. *(Osteoporosis Australia.)*

Why go back to basics?
Because we know there's nothing more frustrating than programmes that ask too much of you, ones that expect you to be able to run for 10 minutes on day one when you know you just can't. Because we know that the last time you ran for the bus, you probably missed it. Because we know runners who were so terrified of exercising in public that they'd run only under the cover of darkness, or jog with a shopping bag so they could pretend they weren't running at all but merely in a rush to get to the supermarket! With this plan, it doesn't matter where you are now or how embarrassed and unfit you feel – you'll definitely be able to manage it. We promise.

So why listen to us?
As fitness journalists, we have access to all the latest running research and the best experts, so we can give you the lowdown on the technical stuff. But that's not all this book is about. The fact is that we're runners ourselves, and we've learned things you can discover only by getting out there and running. Which means that whatever you're going through, we've been there, too.

And because one of us is a tortoise, a slow but sure runner who always gets to the end eventually, and the other a hare who loves tearing after the front runners, we know all about the challenges different types of running bring. Between us, we've made just about every mistake in the book. We know what it's like to shoot out of the door on the first day of your new fitness regime, so overenthusiastic that you attempt to run full-tilt for 20 minutes, only to wilt so badly after ten that you have to catch a taxi home. What it's like to go running in winter in a T-shirt and almost turn blue from the cold.

We know what it is like to be so late for a race that you hear the start gun go off while you're still stuck in the portable loo with your knickers round your ankles. Or to break the biggest rule of all, and run a marathon in spanking new trainers that turn your feet into a bubble wrap of blisters after the first mile.

We've also experienced pretty much every positive emotion running can arouse – the joy of achieving what you set out to do, the deep satisfaction of realising you've been running three times a week for six months and it no longer feels like a struggle, and the pride in finishing a tough race you never thought you could.

Best of all, we're still running and loving every step. We try never to lose sight of the fact that running is fun, and that's why we do it. We know that as well as exercising our glutes, hamstrings and quads, each run should never fail to exercise 53 really important muscles that aren't used nearly often enough – the ones that make you smile!

66 We try never to lose sight of the fact that running is fun, and that's why we do it 99

NINE MIGHTY FINE REASONS TO RUN

1 Because you can indulge in **chocolate** (and other naughty treats) without putting on weight.

2 Because you'll be radiating so much **confidence** your friends will be forced to reach for their sunglasses.

3 Because it will give you the **energy** to bound through your day and still have enough va-va-voom left to shake your thang after 5.30pm.

4 Because it will help **banish cellulite**, which means you'll be able to wear shorts so brief they'd make even Kylie blush.

5 Because the ear-to-ear grin that running gives you will make you totally **irresistible**.

6 Because being successful at running makes you realise you can dare to go after your **dreams** – however wild and crazy they seem.

7 Because it'll make you feel **young** and help you turn back the clock without booking in for Botox.

8 Because you'll get **rich** quick by saving the money you'd have wasted on 'miracle' diet books, faddy low-calorie foods and cigarettes.

9 Because it's so **easy** to fit into your life, it'll leave you plenty of time for shopping, socialising, sangria and sex!

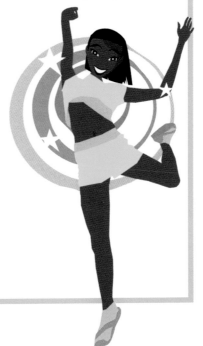

What exactly will I learn?

Basically, how to run. And although it sounds simple, it does need to be learned. Which is where *Running Made Easy* comes in. We want to be with you every step of the way, and that's why this book is packed with all you need to know to help you achieve just about any running goal you might set yourself. We also want it to be really useful, which is why it's also a workbook that we hope you'll fill in regularly to help you track your progress and record your personal achievements, from the joy of going farther than you've ever gone before to the satisfaction of losing that first inch off your hips.

But will it inspire me?

Yes, because you'll find this book is full of tips and advice from ordinary people just like you – and a few extraordinary ones, too, like the 90-year-old marathon addict, the woman who lost half her bodyweight through running and the blind man who still dares to run. You'll learn what motivates people to run, what helps them stick at it when the going gets tough, and hear more about how they came to realise that, by running, they really could change their life for the better. It really is stirring stuff – we were amazed and we think you'll be, too.

  This is also a book that devotes as much time to examining the mental and emotional benefits of running as the physical ones. It'll show you how you can use running as a self-help tool to calm yourself after a frantic day in the office, develop the self-esteem you'll never find at the bottom of a

beer glass, and gain the body confidence that a whole new designer wardrobe can't deliver.

So when do I start?

In a minute! Just one last thing. Always remember that whoever you are, and whatever your starting point, you can be a good runner – it's not about being fast or first, it's about achieving what you set out to do, whether that's one lap of the park, 10 minutes on the treadmill, or finishing your first race or marathon. But most of all, it's about having fun!

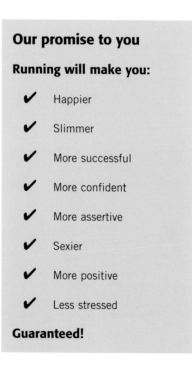

Our promise to you

Running will make you:

✔ Happier

✔ Slimmer

✔ More successful

✔ More confident

✔ More assertive

✔ Sexier

✔ More positive

✔ Less stressed

Guaranteed!

'What I wish I'd known before I started...'

Not everyone gets to read a copy of *Running Made Easy* before embarking on their first run! Here, a few runners share the mistakes they made, to help stop you from making them, too.

'I wish that someone had told me that at the start of every run, I'd have to be patient and wait for my body to warm up. I always set off feeling terrible, and my body would feel like it was shocked because one minute I'd been sitting on the sofa, and the next I was out running. But, if I stuck with it and gave myself time to get into my stride, it started to get a lot easier.'
Jill Hopper, 38, journalist, London

'It's good to plan a running route so you have some idea of where you're going. The first time I ran, I got lost and had to ask people the way home! I got on much better when I found some local running routes on the internet. It also meant I knew exactly how far I was running which helped to motivate me.'
Will Fuller, 35, HR Manager, Surrey

'It took me a while to realise how much easier I'd find it running with someone. I'd get bored and lonely running by myself (music was the only thing that kept me going) but when I was with a friend, I could chat away quite happily which passed the time and meant I didn't really focus on the fact that I was finding it hard work.'
Lindsay Cunningham, 34, teacher, Hampshire

'Running gives you energy when you're tired, and helps you to eat more healthily. As a student nurse, I can be on my feet for 12 hours a day and I used to sometimes think I was too tired to go for a run, so would pick myself up by eating crisps and chocolate instead. But now I've realised that running is a brilliant way to de-stress, and when I've finished a run, I want to eat healthily rather than undo all my good work with junk food.'
Rose Danaher, 27, student nurse, London

'It would have been good to get my underwear sorted earlier on! When I took up running to train for a marathon, I did a few races wearing uncomfortable knickers, and ended up with really sore, chafed legs where the seams had rubbed. I eventually realised the fewer seams the better, and at times I even found it was best to go commando under my shorts!'
Rachel Roberts, 29, teacher, Cornwall

Prepare to see some truly stunning transformations. Each of the ten people overleaf has taken a leap of faith and run their way from fat to fit – gaining heaps of confidence along the way. Between them, they've lost an amazing 326kg (51st 2lb) – and if they can do it, you can, too!

2

get inspired

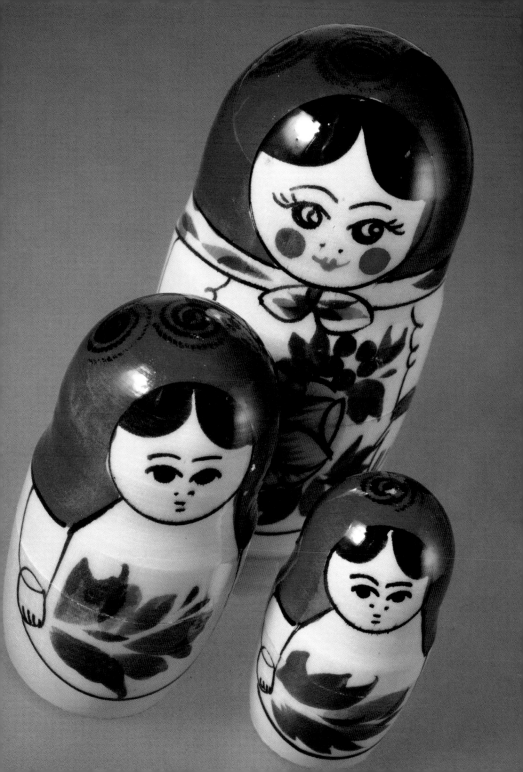

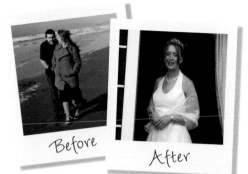

Before

After

Dee Grimes, 31
after-school centre manager
Height 1.73m (5ft 8in)

Before	After
102kg (16st)	70kg (11st)
Dress size 18	Dress size 10/12

✳ **WEIGHT LOST 32kg (5st)**

'RUNNING MADE EASY HELPED ME LOSE FIVE STONE'

❝ I'm a changed woman, thanks to *Running Made Easy*! It helped me go from being overweight and unfit to doing my first marathon in just 18 months. I had a weight problem all my life and as a child was painfully shy. It was a vicious circle. I knew I needed to exercise and slim down but I was too self-conscious to wear workout gear, so I remained overweight. It wasn't food that was the problem – I ate a healthy, vegetarian diet – just the lack of activity.

After I had my first child, Sean, my weight hit an all-time high of 102kg (16st). I felt awful. I hated buying clothes and going out. Three years later, I developed a blood clot in my lung, which made me realise I needed to change my lifestyle. I began to go out for walks and do Pilates and gradually slimmed down to 89kg (14st).

That's when I bought a copy of *Running Made Easy*. It became my bible and I took it everywhere. I liked it so much I read it twice! I embarked on The 60-Second-Secret Plan. Soon afterwards, I signed up for the 10K (6-mile) Women's Mini-Marathon in Dublin. I had a great race and this spurred me on to keep running. And

as I did so, the weight just kept falling off. By the time I got married, I was 70kg (11st).

Over the next year I completed six more races and finished the Dublin Marathon (42.2K/26.2 miles) in 4 hours. I've since had another child and running has helped me regain my pre-pregnancy figure. Before I read *Running Made Easy*, I thought running was only for athletes, but it helped me see that even if you're not super-fast and don't train every day you can still be proud to call yourself a runner. ❞

How Dee did it

Training tip: 'Don't skip your rest days – your body needs them in order to recover from training sessions.'

Motivation tip: 'My motto is "Get up and out!" Don't give yourself time to think before starting an early morning training session – just head for the door and tell yourself you'll do just a few minutes. Once you get going you'll find you're happy to run for much longer than that.'

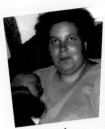

Before

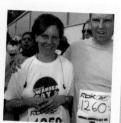

After

Sian Wembridge, 32
Slimming World consultant
Height 1.57m (5ft 2in)

Before	After
143kg (22st 7lb)	60kg (9st 7lb)
Dress size 32	Dress size 8/10

✳ WEIGHT LOST 83kg (13st)

'I LOST 13 STONE – AND KEPT IT OFF WITH RUNNING'

❝ I was a fit and active teenager but then, at the age of 19, I had a miscarriage and tried to overcome my grief through comfort eating. From then on, my weight crept up with every birthday until I weighed 143kg (22st 7lb). My eating habits were appalling. The bigger I got, the less energy I had to cook, and I began to live off takeaways and junk food.

The turning point came when I took my children to Disneyland Paris. I was devastated that I was too heavy to go on some of the rides. A few months later, I finally plucked up the courage to attend a Slimming World meeting. Nineteen months on, I reached 60kg (9st 7lb), having lost 83kg (13st).

When I'd started nearing my goal weight, I'd realised I'd need to exercise to reach my target and also to stop myself regaining the weight afterwards, so I entered a Race For Life and started training. During my first run I thought my lungs would burst, but gradually I started running for longer and I stopped having to walk. I was ecstatic when I finished the 5K (3-mile) race in 39 minutes. After doing two 10K (6-mile) races, I entered the Cardiff half marathon.

When I crossed the finish line in 2 hours and 9 minutes, I sobbed. I couldn't believe that whereas 20 months before I hadn't been able to walk to the end of the street, I'd now run 21K (13.1 miles)!

Running has totally transformed my life. Not only did it enable me to lose the final 6kg (1st) it has helped me keep slim. My daughter Kayleigh loves being able to tell her friends, 'My mummy can run for 13 miles.' And it's the best feeling in the world knowing I can do things I couldn't do before, from cartwheels to simply helping my son Thomas tie his shoes. ❞

How Sian did it

Training tip: 'When I'm doing a 13-mile race, I carry 13 energy tablets with me and have one at every mile marker. It's really motivating feeling my pocket gradually empty!'
Motivation tip: 'Just when your body says it can't go on, remember you can always squeeze in a little bit more, even if it's only 100 yards.'

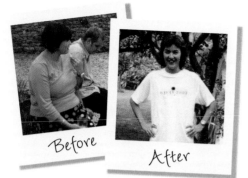

Before

After

Karen Reeve, 28
PA
Height 1.7m (5ft 7in)

Before	**After**
86kg (13st 8lb)	64kg (10st 1lb)
Dress size 18/20	Dress size 12

✳ **WEIGHT LOST 22kg (3st 7lb)**

'I RAN MY WAY INTO A SIZE 12 WEDDING DRESS'

❝ If someone had told me, as I sat crying about the way I looked, that in less than 12 months I'd be 22kg (3st 7lb) slimmer, I wouldn't have believed them. A hideous photo of me taken at my partner Nick's 30th birthday prompted me to get fit. I didn't have the money for a gym, so I opted for running. The day I promised myself I'd start, a storm was raging but I set off regardless. I had to combine small amounts of running with walking because I was so unfit but, despite the weather, it was really exhilarating and I've never looked back.

Nick had proposed to me a short time before I started running, so I used the wedding as an incentive to keep up my new fitness and healthy-eating regime. I lost the weight easily, and each dress fitting reminded me of how far I'd come, making me all the more determined to succeed. By the time I got married, I was overjoyed that I was going to be a slim bride.

I'd always said I was going to go for a run on my wedding day, and I meant it. That morning, I leaped out of bed and opened the presents Nick had given me the night before. My favourite was a personalised T-shirt with a twist! On one side it said the name of our church and our wedding date, and on the reverse it said 'bride'. I ran only 5K (3 miles) that day but I felt really elated. I still smile when I think of all the congratulatory beeps from passing drivers as they read my T-shirt! At the reception Nick made a speech and held up the T-shirt, saying, 'Karen was really determined to go for a run this morning, so I made her this.' It was lovely and everyone gave me a round of applause.

I'm still totally passionate about running and feel I owe a lot to it. Anyone who says they can't run is wrong – just look at me! ❞

How Karen did it
Training tip: 'Follow a training programme – and stick to it. I typed mine up and loved crossing through every run once I'd finished it.'
Motivation tip: 'Give yourself rewards. I had a special nutty cereal that I ate after my weekly 21K (13-mile) route. I really looked forward to it.'

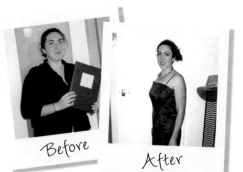

Before

After

Laura Barnes, 26
web project leader
Height 1.63m (5ft 4in)

Before	**After**
89kg (14st)	54kg (8st 7lb)
Dress size 18	Dress size 8/10

✳ WEIGHT LOST 35kg (5st 7lb)

'I CAN DO SO MUCH MORE WITH MY BODY THAN BEFORE'

❝ I put on a lot of weight at university by feasting on tubs of ice cream and drinking lots of gin and tonics, but I found it hard to motivate myself to change my habits and get fit. Although I always knew running would be a brilliant way of losing weight, I felt apprehensive about trying it as I'd always failed at it in the past. I also really worried about people seeing the colour my face went on a run. But then a truly awful photo of me looking podgy-faced and piggy-eyed finally motivated me to start losing weight.

After about 13kg (2st) had come off, I entered a 5K (3-mile) race with three friends – I loved the fact that it was an all-women run because it felt really non-competitive. Having something like that looming meant I had to start training, so I set off with a friend, doing just 30 seconds at a time with lots of walking in between. We were amazed at how fast we built up to running 8K (5 miles), and even had enough puff left to talk the whole time! I found race day terrifying, but the four of us ran together until competition got the better of us and I won the sprint for the finish line!

Running got me fitter than anything else I'd ever tried, and helped me lose more weight than I'd ever thought possible – a total of 35kg (5st 7lb). My appearance changed so much that the compliments started to flood in and even my own mum once walked past me without recognising me!

The experience also completely transformed my view of what I'm capable of. Something I feared has now become something I love. I even keep my race medal on view to remind me of my achievements. I've realised I can do much more with my body than before. Now, instead of sitting at work feeling big and miserable, I sit there itching to get outside and run. ❞

How Laura did it
Training tip: 'I don't tell myself I have to run for a certain time or distance – sometimes I literally just go round the block, which takes only 4 minutes.'
Motivation tip: 'Running along chatting with a friend made even 6.5K (4-mile) runs fun and helped them to pass more quickly.'

23

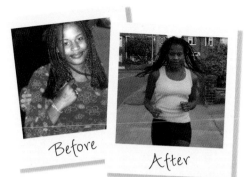

Before

After

Teba Diatta, 22
journalism student
Height 1.63m (5ft 4in)

Before	After
73kg (11st 7lb)	57kg (9st)
Dress size 14/16	Dress size 10

✱ **WEIGHT LOST 16kg (2st 7lb)**

'RUNNING RESTORED MY BODY CONFIDENCE'

❝ I took up running aged 18 and was a fit and healthy size 10 by the time I decided to spend my gap year in Senegal teaching in a village school. My British mother met my Senegalese father there when she went to West Africa as a missionary, and I'd always been curious to meet my extended family. I continued running in Senegal, gradually building up to being able to run for miles from village to village in the fierce African sun. When I got back to the UK, however, I had to stop exercising completely while recovering from an operation, and almost before I knew it, comfort eating whole packets of chocolate biscuits in one sitting had resulted in me putting on 16kg (2st 7lb). I felt awful and my confidence totally evaporated. I started university but felt so self-conscious that I didn't enjoy meeting new people.

After failing at a long succession of diets, I eventually joined a gym and started running again. I was shocked at how hard even 5 minutes of running had become, but I kept going, spurred on by the way the pounds were melting away. I was thrilled when, after six months, I reached my current weight of 57kg (9st).

I knew I wanted to do something with my new fitness and resolved to run 320K (200 miles) from York Minster cathedral in York to Westminster Abbey in London to raise money to buy equipment for the Senegalese school I'd taught in. I ran for 18 days – at one point I ran a half-marathon every day for six days. To keep me motivated I thought of the children in Senegal who ran alongside me for miles in their flip-flops. I hope the money I've raised will mean the next time I go running with them, they'll be wearing trainers. ❞

How Teba did it

Training tip: 'Don't go too fast, too soon. I find the treadmill is really useful for building up your speed in small stages.'

Motivation tip: 'Having seen lots of children in Senegal walk tens of miles a day to and from school, I know the true meaning of the expression, "Where there's a will, there's a way." I believe that if you sort out your mind, your body will follow.'

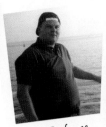

Before

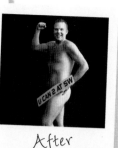

After

David Howard, 31
motor mechanic
Height 1.83m (6ft)

Before	**After**
130kg (20st 6lb)	89kg (14st)
Waist size	Waist size
107cm (42in)	91cm (36in)

✱ WEIGHT LOST 41kg (6st 6lb)

'I LOST MY SPARE TYRE – AND BECAME A PIN-UP!'

66 Drinking 15 to 20 pints of beer three nights a week – plus eating a few too many kebabs and burgers – meant I went from a big lad of 108kg (17st) when I left school to an even bigger one in my twenties. For ten years I weighed 130kg (20st 6lb). Then one January I resolved to slim down after getting my enormous belly stuck under a trailer at work! In the same week I joined a gym and Slimming World diet club, as I'd never tried to lose weight before and felt I needed some advice.

At the first few sessions, I could manage only a 5-minute walk on the treadmill before I had to sit down. But after a few weeks, I tried a gentle jog and I gradually progressed from there. I soon got tired of indoor running and began running outside, which I much preferred. By March, I'd built up to running 14.4K (9 miles) several times a week and in just 18 weeks I lost a whopping 41kg (6st 6lb)! Sticking to the Slimming World programme so religiously was key to my success, but I soon realised it was vital to combine it with running. In the weeks when I ran, I lost about 4kg (9lb), but in those when I didn't, I lost only 1kg (2lb).

I really love the new me. It's great walking to the shops without getting out of breath, and being able to play football. Losing weight also had another unexpected result: *Slimming World Magazine* asked me to pose for their calendar – in the nude! I agreed as I thought my weight loss might inspire other people. Sometimes I can't believe that fit-looking man is really me. My mum bought 20 copies of the calendar and I even have one on the wall at the garage where I work. Who would ever have guessed that I'd become a pin-up? **99**

How David did it

Eating tip: 'Never ever run on a full stomach. I tried it once and ran for 3K (2 miles) before being struck down with an agonising stitch.'

Motivation tip: 'Talk to other runners when you're out training – you'll be amazed how friendly they can be. I've met loads of interesting people through running and enjoyed some top nights out with them.'

Photograph by Bill Morton courtesy of *Slimming World Magazine*

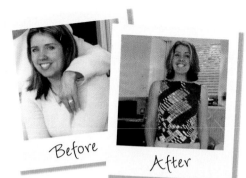

Before

After

Shonagh Woods, 34
marketing manager
Height 1.68m (5ft 6in)

Before	After
79kg (12st 6lb)	60kg (9st 6lb)
Dress size 14/16	Dress size 10

✳ WEIGHT LOST 19kg (3st)

'RUNNING IS GOOD FOR BODY AND SOUL!'

❝ When I started bulging out of my size 14 clothes but couldn't bear to buy a size 16, I knew I had to do something about my weight. I felt as if the real me was hiding inside the body of a fat person and couldn't get out. Things changed when I got engaged and realised I had to lose the weight fast for my wedding. I simply couldn't bear the idea of being a fat bride, and the thought of my future children looking at my fat wedding photos filled me with horror.

I wasn't sure where to start until my best friend bought me a brilliant book on running for Christmas. I'd always thought of running as boring but the book really inspired me. There was a long, straight road where I lived, and I'd set off running along it for 5 minutes then run back for five.

When I was able to run for 10 minutes out and 10 back, I hopped in the car to measure the distance and was ecstatic to find I could run 3K (2 miles)! I found the running was not only making me lose weight – about 3kg (7lb) a month – but was good for my soul, too. I started feeling I was back in control of my life again. Muscles were appearing in my legs and along the sides of my stomach where I'd never known they existed, and my jeans became too big.

On my wedding day I was 13kg (2st) lighter and felt brilliant – there wasn't a single photo I didn't like. But things have got even better since. I went on to run my first half-marathon (21K/13.1miles) and at 60kg (9st 6lb) I'm now down to my slimmest ever. I also feel amazingly positive about other things in life that I might once have doubted I could do, be or say. Because I started from scratch and transformed myself into a runner, I now believe I can achieve whatever I want. ❞

How Shonagh did it

Training tip: 'Don't think you can't run – just get yourself a good pair of trainers and then set off really slowly.'

Motivation tip: 'Realise what running can do for your mind. I always come back from a run feeling a lot less stressed, full of ideas and with solutions to my problems.'

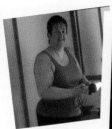

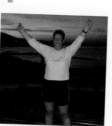

Before

After

Gill Kelley, 49
management trainer
Height 1.65m (5ft 5in)

Before
103kg (16st 3lb)
Dress size 22

After
86kg (13st 8lb)
Dress size 18

✳ WEIGHT LOST 17kg (2st 9lb)

'RUNNING HAD AN AMAZING EFFECT ON MY BODY'

66 A diet of pork pies and crisps bought from motorway service stations was the reason I became overweight almost without noticing it. One day I realised that if I wanted to be fit enough to enjoy early retirement, I'd better get my skates on.

I was careful not to overdo it at first, so I jogged from one lamp-post to the next, then walked for two lamp-posts, and so on. I found it really hard early on and I wish someone had told me before I started that the first kilometre or mile is always difficult – but after that it gets much easier.

I persevered with my lamp-posts and before long built up to running for 30 minutes each day before work. I loved the adrenaline buzz it gave me. The effects on my body were amazing – in the first few months, I lost up to 1.5kg (3lb) each week. In just under a year, I lost 17kg (2st 9lb) and felt better than I had done in years. I'm not at my goal weight yet but I know I'll reach it eventually. My fitness progress also amazed me: soon after I'd started running, I managed a 5K (3-mile) race and three months later, I surprised myself by completing a half-marathon.

I've always wanted to say I'd done a marathon before the age of 50 – but never really wanted to actually run one! With only 18 months to go before turning 50, I plucked up the courage to run the Flora London Marathon for Shelter, a homelessness charity. It was a very hot day but I felt brilliant the whole way and was amazed at what my body was capable of. I raised £1,500 and that really helped get me through the race – I knew I just had to finish. You should have seen the grin on my face in the photo of me at the halfway mark, and when I crossed the finish line after 7 hours and 15 minutes! **99**

How Gill did it
Training tip: 'Run with your dog – I love running with mine along the canal paths near my home.'
Motivation tip: 'Always try to turn negatives into positives. When my legs are aching at the start of a run, I tell myself that carrying on running until my muscles are warm will make them feel better.'

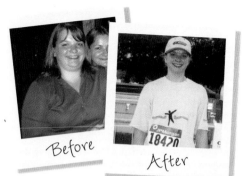

Before

After

Julie McWhirr, 27
investment banker
Height 1.63m (5ft 4in)

Before	After
94kg (14st 11lb)	66kg (10st 6lb)
Dress size 20	Dress size 12

✳ **WEIGHT LOST 28kg (4st 5lb)**

'I THOUGHT I WAS DESTINED TO BE FAT FOR EVER'

❝ The crunch came when I was out shopping for a special outfit. I'd convinced myself I looked OK in the size 20 dress I was trying on, until I found myself in front of the communal mirror next to a size 10 girl trying on the same dress! I realised then that I had to do something about the ridiculous amount of weight I'd put on, so when a friend joined Weight Watchers, I followed suit. After I'd lost the first 4.5kg (10lb), I started to exercise gently by walking on a treadmill. I'm a determined person with lots of willpower, so I stuck at it until I could gradually turn up the speed and start running. After each run, I started to feel a high I'd never experienced before. And the more weight I lost, the more confidence I had to do new things, like join an all-women running club (called The Epsom Allsorts because it's a real mix of people, from girls to grandmas!).

The weight kept falling off steadily, while the running started to tone me. I was also developing collarbones – it's such a novelty to have them there! But the best thing about running was that it kept me positive and gave me a non-weight-related goal that stopped the

weigh-in at Weight Watchers dictating my whole mood for the week. In fact, by the time I'd reached my goal weight of 66kg (10st 6lb), I had another, more important goal in mind – to run a half-marathon (21K/13.1 miles).

The race was incredible! I loved every minute of it and kept slowing down because I wanted it to last longer. I always thought I was destined to be fat for the rest of my life – these days, I often walk past shop windows and don't recognise myself. And I know that by keeping on running, I'll stay this way for good. ❞

How Julie did it
Motivation tip: 'If I ever lack motivation, I ask my partner Ian to give me three good reasons why I should go for a run. By the time he's listed them, I'm up off the sofa and out of the front door.'
Eating tip: 'Even if you're trying to lose weight, you do need to eat enough to give you the energy to run. Don't expect to go out and run for miles on a diet of salad and apples alone.'

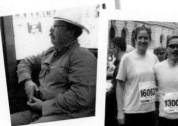
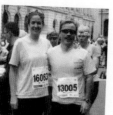

Before

After

Billy Pearce, 39
nurse manager
Height 1.7m (5ft 7in)

Before	**After**
106kg (16st 10lb)	73kg (11st 7lb)
Waist size	Waist size
112cm (44in)	81cm (32in)

✳ WEIGHT LOST 33kg (5st 3lb)

'I'VE RUN MY WAY TO A HEALTHY HEART'

❝ My real weight problems started in my early thirties when I worked as an overland safari guide in Africa. I'd sit on my backside all day in the truck and overindulge in fatty food. Exercise was the last thing on my mind, and at my heaviest I weighed 106kg (16st 10lb). While my appearance didn't bother me, I did want to get healthy by the time I was 40, as my dad had died prematurely of heart disease and I didn't want to follow in his footsteps.

I decided to lose weight when my wife and I were upgraded on our flight home after our honeymoon. Instead of tucking into the wine and chocolates, I just felt sick of it all, and decided to start a healthy-eating plan. I also began running at the gym. I didn't enjoy it but stuck at it through sheer bloody-mindedness.

Things improved when I joined a running club and began to run outdoors. Within two years I'd lost 33kg (5st 3lb) and started training for the Flora London Marathon (42K/26.2 miles). I was picked to join the team of Nike Bowerman runners, a group of normal runners that Nike supports and gives expert help to. They did lots of tests on me, which helped me see how

my heart rate was slowing and my cholesterol levels were dropping as I became fitter, which kept me motivated. I'm happy with the way my body has changed and feel much more confident about buying clothes or going swimming. But most of all I love the way I feel, and that I know my heart is fit and healthy, too.

I completed the London Marathon in 4 hours and 10 minutes, and now I'm helping encourage new runners to join our running club. Life is good – and I want more of that. ❞

How Billy did it
Motivation tip: 'Don't just think about what running can do for your appearance – be aware of what it's doing for your health, too. For added motivation, try tracking not just the weight you're losing but your heart rate, which will slow as you get fitter.'
Eating tip: 'I don't need to stick to a diet – I just make sure I never have too much fat, which means I can eat a little of whatever I want.'

○ ○ ○ Do you want to wake up happy every day and bounce through life with a permanent smile on your face? All it takes to feel this good is something that gets your mind as fit as your body – we recommend a regular dose of running…

3

get happy

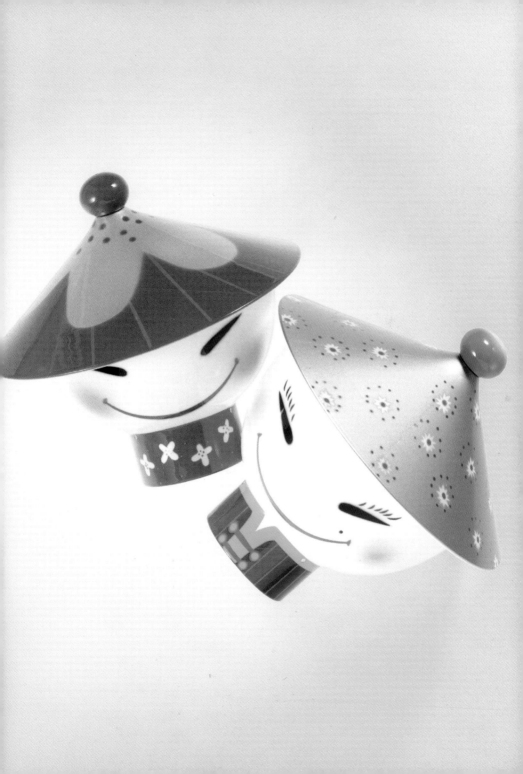

How happy do you feel? Could you be happier? Would you love to learn to laugh your way through every day? If the answer's yes, then running is a brilliant way to increase your happiness potential, pretty much overnight.

So why does running have such a profound effect on what's going on in your head? According to a study conducted at the University of Missouri-Columbia, USA, the four key ingredients you need to feel happy and content are as follows:

✔ self-esteem
✔ a sense of control
✔ a feeling of competence
✔ feeling connected to others

And running delivers on every single one of them. Here's how...

1 How running builds your self-esteem

Talk to any runner and they'll tell you that their self-esteem has soared since they took up running. Of course, this is partly to do with becoming the proud owner of a fit and healthy body, capable of doing things you once only dreamed of, but it's also about demonstrating to yourself, and other people, that you can move mountains if you set your mind to it.

'When I scaled back my teaching job to spend more time with my three daughters, I found there's not much status in being a housewife and a mum,' says runner and mother of three Fiona Lunskey, 38. 'Taking up running and telling people that I was going to run a 5K (3-mile) race has given me something to feel proud of. Even though it's not as if your name is up in lights for doing a race, that's what it feels like to you. And my daughters started talking about their mummy as a runner, which I felt good about – I wanted to show them it's not just daddies who are sporty while mummies cook and clean, but that mummies can put on their trainers and achieve things, too.' Of course, the fact that you feel like a celebrity during races – when thousands of people are clapping for you and shouting your name – doesn't hurt either!

2 How running gives you a sense of control

Unlike team sports or classes at the gym, where you have to grit your teeth for a solid 45 minutes, you're always the one who's in charge. You get to decide exactly when you'll run – on your way to work, in that 30-minute slot that unexpectedly opened up in your diary or before heading out for a night on the town with your mates. You get to decide how far you'll go – up the road, round the park, or until you've had enough. And you get to set the pace – whether it's a leisurely sightseeing trot or a faster-than-a-speeding-bullet gallop.

When you're a beginner, there's no need to lurk at the back of a class, hoping you won't attract the attention of the gym instructor while praying for the 45 minutes to be over – you simply go at your own speed and do your own thing for as long as you like.

You're the boss! And as you start to achieve your goals, that feeling of control just grows and grows.

3 How running makes you feel competent

Succeeding at a physical activity like running teaches you about all those hidden abilities you never realised you had. Daring, and managing, to run a lap of the park, or even a race, will give you the confidence to stick your hand in the air and say, 'I can do that!' about all sorts of other things you might never have even tried. 'After I ran the New York City Marathon, I felt I could have done anything – gone off and climbed Mount Everest, whatever!' says Shelly Vella, 37, fashion director of British *Cosmopolitan*. Other people swear that they can channel the feelings of competence they get from running to help them through difficult situations. One runner who was struggling in her new job and feeling out of her depth

discovered that by going off and running at the gym at lunchtime she was able to come back into those intimidating afternoon meetings and face her boss feeling in control and able to cope.

4 How running makes you feel connected to other people

Become a runner and you instantly become part of an amazingly diverse, worldwide community of millions of people all interested in the same thing. From chief executives and film stars to Kenyans who run miles and miles to school every day, and bikini-clad babes who strut their stuff beachside in LA, you'll find so many different people who run and with whom you've got an instant bond.

And, if you start taking part in races and events, you'll find the bond grows even stronger. As David Traub, 56, a solicitor from Johannesburg, South Africa, puts it, 'Running is special because in other sports you just don't get the same camaraderie with your opponents. I think this is because your opponent isn't the person next to you, it's the road itself. Of course, you want to do your best, but at the same time you want everyone else to do well, too.' And few things can make you feel closer to other people than sharing the same experiences, overcoming the same challenges and finally dissolving into tears of joy as you all cross that finish line together.

Get ready for more good news

Now you've got those four fab happiness ingredients firmly fixed in your mind, you're well on your way to the happiest-ever you. But the story doesn't end there…

Running gets you buzzing

This is all thanks to the streams of lovely endorphins that flow around your body when you run, and which help to produce a top-of-the-world feeling often called the 'runner's high'. Endorphins are actually hormones that are secreted from your brain in response to a variety of stimuli, including exercise, and that are 100 to 200 times more powerful than morphine, the most powerful drug used in hospitals! 'Even though the release of endorphins is quite short-lived, the feeling of being on a high can go on for hours,' says endocrinologist Professor Nadir Farid from private hospital The London Clinic. 'One theory is that this is because the release of endorphins triggers a kind of chain reaction in your body, which then keeps you feeling good long term.' Another great thing is that endorphins aren't shy or elusive – most people who run experience this feel-good buzz. In fact, in one study, 85% of people said they felt a natural high from exercising, which lasted anywhere between a few hours and all day or night!

It gets you loving

The fitter you are, the better your circulation becomes, which ensures you have a good supply of blood to keep those vital organs (and we're not talking heart and brain here!) working perfectly. Couple this with the fact that once you've taken up running, your body image and self-esteem improve, and it's no wonder that fit people are more likely than couch potatoes to be in the mood for love. Almost a third of members of Cannons health clubs questioned as part of a Mind survey said their sex drive had improved since they'd taken up exercise, while more than half said their general relationship with their partner had markedly improved.

It gets you thinking

Whether you're trying to solve a niggling problem, survive a tricky situation, come up with a bright idea, or simply get away from it all and relax, running seems to have an uncanny ability to lead you to what you

HOT DATE 1 MILE

need. It's as if once you've struck up the right rhythm and breathing pattern, your mind is set free to wander, which is why so many fans refer to their running as a form of meditation or therapy. 'I don't set off on a run thinking I have to work through what's worrying me,' says Jennie Francis, 45, a hypnotherapist from London, 'but if I've got a problem or something I'm putting off, by the time I finish my run and have a shower it doesn't feel like such a big deal. Both the breathing and the repetitive action of running are really soothing. I've studied lots of complementary therapies, and I'd compare the effect that running has to getting into a meditative state.'

It gets you feeling at one with the world

Think about how much time you spend outdoors every day and, unless you're quite exceptional, it's probably just a few minutes on the way between the office and the car or train, and maybe a little potter around your garden when you get home. Running gives you a reason to get outside, opens up new horizons, and even helps fulfil our basic need to feel at one with nature – something that's known as biophilia. Studies have been done that show that meeting this basic need can boost happiness and even help people heal faster after operations and traumas. You'll also see and experience things that other people miss (from the ducklings on your local pond to the wafting smells of people's Sunday dinners cooking!). 'I tend to feel more down in the winter because I really miss the sunshine and find it hard to get outdoors,' says Nicola Cawley, 29,

a lawyer from Buckinghamshire. 'That all changed when I started training for the Flora London Marathon and was outside running in all weathers. Although it felt strange at first, I realised I was enjoying getting all that fresh air and daylight every day.'

It gets you through the hard times

Running doesn't just make happy people happier. It's also great for helping you out in your hour of need, whether you're depressed or just stressed. A study published in the *British Journal of Sports Medicine* found exercise may be more effective than drugs at treating mild to moderate depression. In the study doing just 30 minutes of exercise a day significantly improved the mood of patients who'd been suffering from depression for nine months. Another study carried out on people with mental health problems found 65% of them felt exercise had helped to relieve the symptoms of depression. For more proof of running's ability to combat depression – and instil calm and confidence – turn the page...

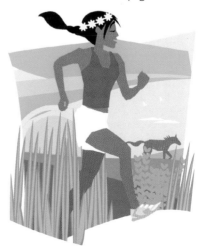

'We ran our way back to happiness'

'Running helped me through the worst time in my life'
Peter Greene, 42, negotiator, London

❝I used to be a good cross-country runner at school, and I loved the feeling of racing along, knee-deep in mud. I carried on running after school, not only because it made me feel good physically, but also because it helped me cope with my stressful job. I felt my runs set me up for each day, and I'd get a warm glow as the endorphins kicked in.

When I was 39, my younger brother committed suicide. Losing him was a complete shock. I knew he'd been feeling a bit down, but no one in my family realised to what extent.

hit by depression
I experienced my first-ever bout of depression and started to feel really numb and unable to cope with anything. Before my brother's death, my personality had been what I'd call 'Teflon-coated'. I was easy-going and light-hearted and didn't let anything bother me. But when something like a suicide happens, it just shocks you to the core. Problems with my wife started to come to the surface because I became more needy, and my marriage began to break up. My feelings really came out while I was running – I'd run with tears streaming down my face.

clarity and comfort
I went on the antidepressant Prozac, but I felt as if it was closing my mind down. My head felt incredibly cloudy, whereas running had the opposite effect on me. It helped me think straight and understand what was happening to me. I found I could make sense of things on my run.

escape route
Knowing I was going to get up and run first thing in the morning was like an escape for me when everything around me felt as if it was going wrong. Because running is a very determined act – when you're running up a hill, you really have to grit your teeth to get to the top – it also helped me be determined about what I was going to have to do, which was leave my children, my wife and my home.

During the divorce proceedings I carried on running and it kept me going. I'm no longer depressed and I feel as if I've come out of the whole episode with very high self-awareness, knowing how to look after myself. I've come off the Prozac and I feel like myself again. It's nice to be back. **❞**

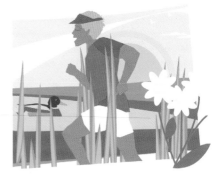

'Running changed me into a can-do person'
Jo Nicolson, 33, photographer, York

❝Just one year ago, I was in a terrible, paranoid state, suffering from such bad anxiety and stress that I had to have time off work. I'd become absolutely convinced I wasn't good enough at my job (working as a photographer for the Royal Air Force) and was going to be sacked at any minute. I was being physically sick during the day and not sleeping at night, my mental capacity had gone down to absolute zero, and it's a miracle I could even drive a car.

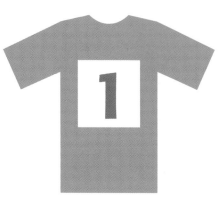

getting help
I started having therapy, which taught me to change my perspective on life, and my therapist suggested I set myself a goal to help motivate me and raise my self-esteem. I chose to run the Flora London Marathon for Shelter, a charity for the homeless. I'd always run to keep fit, and was dead keen to do the marathon, but I had held back because a little voice in my head kept telling me I wouldn't make it. But, thanks to the therapy, I started to feel, 'Actually, I can do it.'

fast track to feel-good
Once I started running with the marathon as a goal, it dramatically changed my mental state. Just the fact that I'd got up and been for a run instead of sitting on the sofa eating biscuits made such a difference to the rest of my day, and I'd come back feeling refreshed. It gave me a break from endlessly mulling over my problems in my head, and it gave my partner a break from having to listen to me! Running became like my meditation, when I could really switch off and relax, and it felt as restful as having a lovely sleep. It worked hand in hand with the therapy I was having to restore my self-esteem and rebuild my confidence.

When I ran the marathon, it was phenomenal, everything I'd ever dreamed it would be. I started crying at 32K (20 miles) because I was so pleased I was going to make it, and carried on crying for the next 10K (6 miles)! I was so elated when I went into work the next day because I'd taken the risk and succeeded. I feel as if I've now got so much positive momentum that I can't stop moving forwards. I'm ready to take on the next challenge. All I can think is, where can I go next with this? ❞

'How running makes me feel'

We challenged these runners to capture in words the mood-boosting, grin-inducing power of running...

❝ Ten minutes into a run, a feeling comes over me and **suddenly I'm on a bit of a high and the world seems a better place**. I begin to notice my surroundings more, I look at the clouds and the waves coming in and I feel as if I'm **communing with nature** and that all my everyday cares and concerns are very far away.' Caroline Yarnell, 43, postgraduate student, Sydney, Australia

'I love running because wherever you are in the world, and however you felt before you went for a run, it always has the same effect. Once you've been running, **you feel like a different and better person**. The problem that was nagging away at you has been solved. The sluggishness brought on by jet lag has evaporated, the anger and irritation left behind. Running – always the solution, never the problem.' Marcus Leaver, 33, CEO, London

'When I go out running in the early morning, I'm overcome by the most **intense feeling of peace** and never cease to be amazed at the beauty of my surroundings. Not only do **I feel incredibly alive**, but somehow my feelings of gratitude, for all I have and am able to experience, are enhanced. Experiencing this joy of running is a very special part of my day.'
Anni Walls, 34, entrepreneur, Pretoria, South Africa

'I've been amazed by how much better I feel for running after the birth of my son. Around the time he turned one, I gingerly donned my trainers and set off at tortoise pace. Now I run about three times a week once he's in bed. Even when I'm tired, it picks me up, makes me feel better about my body shape and reminds me I'm still my own person as well as a mum!'
Jill Hopper, 38, journalist, London

'Running gives me a terrific **sense of achievement** and makes me feel alive, even when my lungs are straining and my legs are exhausted. And because it forces me to leave behind modern distractions like mobile phones and TV, it's also one of the best ways to see the world around me and to **reflect on what I'm doing and where I'm going**. Running is exclusively my time – and that's a very rare commodity.' Dan Waugh, 30, corporate affairs manager, London

'One wet lunchtime, I very reluctantly headed off for a run round a park near my office. In fact, it was such a miserable day that I almost turned back when I stepped out into the rain. But by the time I reached the park, the clouds had rolled away and I was greeted by **one of the most awe-inspiring sights I've ever seen**. Every single blade of grass was topped by a glittering raindrop, and in the sunlight all the lawns looked as if they'd had armloads of diamonds scattered over them. I had the whole park to myself and felt almost **overwhelmed by a feeling of gratitude** that running had enabled me to witness such a magical, almost spiritual, moment.' Melanie Calvin, 29, travel PR, Chicago, USA

'Running is **like going into your own private room**. I do my best thinking when I'm running because it really helps clear my mind.'
Alan Nurse, 34, solicitor, London

'I don't have to run every day to be a runner. I don't even have to run every week. Somehow, the act of running has been hardwired into my psyche, and **I'll always be a runner, no matter how irregularly I pound the pavements**. My body is proof of that. I can go for six whole months without putting on my trainers, but the next time I do, my legs will pump obligingly into action, my lungs will spring back to life and my feet will carry me as far as I want to go. It will hurt, but it will happen. My body tells me that even when I'm feeling sad and slow, there is a part of me that will always be strong, and fast, and brave.'
Alexandra Friend, 29, journalist, London

'**The joy of being alive** in the small hours of a sparkling, clear morning, and running amid idyllic landscapes of cool green forests, pastoral valleys, mountain scenery and glistening coastlines is the main reason I love running as much as I do.' Ginette Flockton, 55, teacher, Cape Town, South Africa

'When I moved from South Africa to Winnipeg in Canada, which gets down to an unbelievable -40°C (-40°F), running outside in the winter months didn't seem like an option! However, while running in a windowless basement gym, I was eventually persuaded by a concerned fellow runner to ditch running on the dreadmill (!) and give outdoor running a go. On my first outing **I felt sheer joy** as I raced across the frozen, snow-covered Assiniboine River. Now I run every day in the most beautiful place I've ever run in!
Bridget Robinson, 36, project manager, Winnipeg, Canada 99

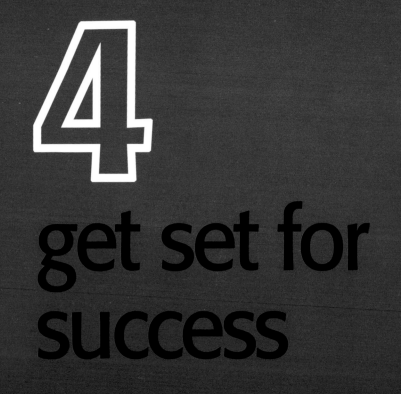

Walt Disney once said, 'If you can dream it, you can do it!' This chapter is your chance to dream – and achieve any goal you've set your heart on…

4

get set for success

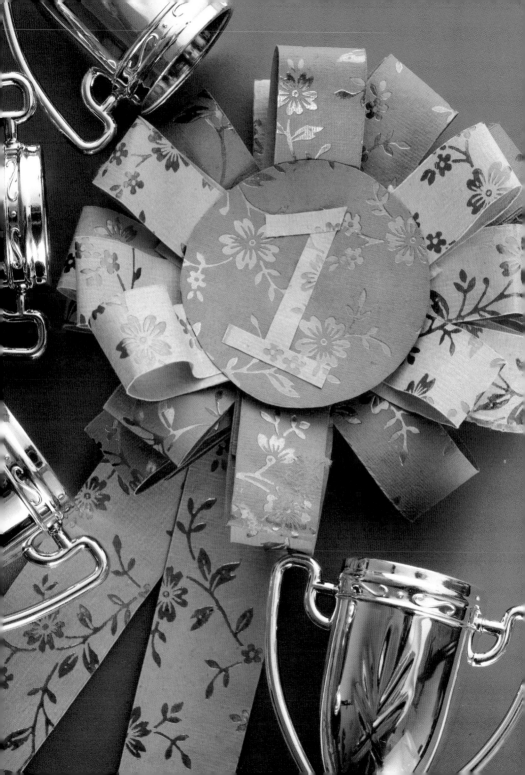

Rather like window-shopping, when you're not actually intending to buy anything and just want to see what's out there, running along without any real purpose can be great fun. But running with a goal in mind can be even better – just as window-shopping becomes more exciting when you spot your perfect pair of designer shoes and know you'll do anything to afford them. Another reason why having something to aim for is important is that experts say 'progressively achieving worthwhile goals' can actually make you happy. So prepare to feel fantastic, because running is unbeatable at providing you with limitless goal-setting opportunities. It's progressive, too, as the training plans you to follow (see Chapters Six and Eight) will help you achieve these goals one step at a time. And, of course, it goes without saying that these goals are incredibly worth while – achieving them will turbo-boost your vitality, your health, your self-image and your mood.

Six steps to success

How do you go about reaching your goals? It's not as difficult as you may have feared. Basically, you can break it all down into six simple steps:

1 Choose your goal

When you're casting about for a goal, remember that, as one author once put it, 'Goals are dreams with deadlines.' Goal-setting simply involves finding out what your dreams really are – and then setting about making them happen within a set time-frame.

Let's do some dreaming right now. First take a look at the Why I Want To Get Fit list (see opposite), which gives you some ideas to get you started, plus space to add your own at the bottom of the page. Then, for the next five minutes, close your eyes and dream the impossible dream, which,

we promise, will become the possible dream sooner than you think. How would you like to look in six months' time? How would you like to feel? What would you like to have accomplished? The kind of goal you should be thinking of should really excite you and give you butterflies in your stomach and shivers down your spine.

Dare to dream big – and don't think to yourself,

WHY I WANT TO GET FIT

✓ I want to love myself more, but have less of me to love.
✓ I want to be able to put all my photos in my albums – not just the ones where my double chin isn't showing.
✓ I want people to say, 'You're looking well' and know that they really mean, 'Wow, you've lost weight!'
✓ I want to banish the blues.
✓ I want to be able to raid my slimmer sister's or brother's wardrobe.
✓ I want to keep up with my hyperactive kids.
✓ I want to shop for head-turning clothes rather than live in saggy tracksuit bottoms and baggy jumpers.
✓ I want to be able to do a 5K (3-mile) fun run with my friends – and actually have fun doing it.
✓ I want to quit smoking.
✓ I want to attend my school reunion and still be able to fit into the blazer I wore when I left school.
✓ I want to be able to race up stairs – and positively bound up escalators without breaking into a sweat.
✓ I want to feel young again.
✓ I want to run a race in a fairy outfit.
✓ I want to take my stress out on the street, not on my partner or my dog.
✓ I want to send my self-esteem rocketing.
✓ I want to boost my chances of getting a telegram from the Queen on my 100th birthday.
✓ I want to banish my beer belly for good and stop letting out notches on my belt.
✓ I want to be smelling the daisies when I'm old – not pushing them up.
✓ I want to boost my mood – without overdosing on chocolate.
✓ I want to say 'I've run a marathon' and tick it off my 'to do' list.
✓ I want to win medals without joining the army.
✓ I want to spend quality time getting to know the real me.
✓ I want to _____
✓ I want to _____
✓ I want to _____
✓ I want to _____
✓ I want to _____
✓ I want to _____
✓ I want to _____

'I'd love to run a 5K (3-mile) race but I'll have to wait until I'm slimmer/fitter/have more time/have given up smoking', as by doing that you're placing limits on what you can achieve. Just as no one can make you feel inferior without your consent (as the USA First Lady Eleanor Roosevelt famously said), no one can put limits on what you can achieve without your permission either. 'I now realise the limits I set for myself were just excuses and that I can do anything, and go as far as I want to go,' says Catherine Mokwena, 41, a South African runner who ran the New York City Marathon with an artificial leg. So even if you're really overweight, desperately out of shape, manically busy and a 20-a-day smoker, just set your goal and leave worrying about how you're going to achieve it to us!

Now write your long-term dream goal into your Mission Statement, which you'll find on page 47.

2 Make sure it's a SMART goal

SMART goals are successful goals. The acronym SMART stands for:

Specific Being very precise about what you want to achieve will give you something tangible to aim for – an example of a specific goal is saying, 'I want to run a 5K (3-mile) race in three months' time dressed as a superhero.' An example of a non-specific goal would simply be saying, 'I want to get fit.'

Measurable This will enable you to know when you've succeeded – which means it's time to celebrate! A good example of a measurable goal would be saying, 'I want to be 13kg (2st)

lighter a year from now and be able to fit into my favourite pair of jeans.'

Achievable Be honest with yourself about your abilities and don't set yourself up for failure by deciding on goals that are totally out of reach (but don't let this stop you dreaming big!). So, while aiming to win your first-ever race may be unrealistic, vowing to come in the top half of the field may be well within your grasp.

Reward-orientated Plan an mmm-I-deserve-this treat for every time you achieve your goals to reinforce your good behaviour and encourage you to keep going.

Time-framed Giving yourself a deadline will provide a sense of urgency – and make you all the more likely to succeed.

3 Break it into bite-sized chunks

Next, set a date for when you want to achieve your goal by and write it into your Mission Statement (see page 47). Then chop it into easily digestible (and doable) chunks. Breaking down a long-term goal into lots of short-term goals you know you're capable of achieving is the key to success. This is often tricky, so you'll be relieved we've already done all the hard work and set out a ten-week step-by-step programme called The 60-Second-Secret Plan for you to follow (see Chapter Six).

4 Work out your rewards

Now it's time for the fun part! Look at the Daily Rewards, Weekly Treats and Ultimate Indulgences (see opposite) for some ideas on how you can reward yourself for all your hard work and commitment.

DAILY REWARDS
★ Read a magazine for half an hour.
★ Savour an ice-cold beer.
★ Wallow in a bubble bath.
★ Eat a healthy treat such as melon, strawberries, lychees or passion fruit.
★ Snooze on the sofa for 30 minutes.
★ Spend 10 minutes in your garden smelling the roses.
★ Read a chapter of a gripping novel.
★ Phone a friend for a chat.
★ Watch some great TV.
★ Spend 10 minutes in the sauna or steam room at your gym.

WEEKLY TREATS
★ Buy a figure-flattering piece of fit kit.
★ Subscribe to an inspiring health or fitness magazine such as *Zest*.
★ Buy a funny book.
★ Have a pampering home spa session in your bathroom.
★ Go out for a slap-up meal.
★ Go to see a great new film.
★ Treat yourself to a healthy brunch.
★ Have a night on the tiles.
★ Rent a must-see DVD.
★ Get that lipstick/handbag/pair of trainers you've had your eye on.

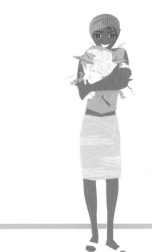

★ Buy a big bouquet of fresh flowers.
★ Spend an evening in front of the fire with a bottle of good wine.
★ Laugh yourself silly at a comedy club.
★ Go on a date with your partner.
★ Go wild at a pop concert.

ULTIMATE INDULGENCES
★ Buy that fab new outfit you've been coveting.
★ Do something crazily exciting like skydiving or bungee-jumping.
★ Be a culture vulture by going to the ballet, opera or a classical concert.
★ Sign up for a course in something you've always dreamed of doing: scuba-diving, wine-tasting, yoga or Indian head massage.
★ Treat yourself to a gym membership.
★ Have an adventurous new haircut.
★ Snare tickets to a glamorous sporting event such as a day at the races, a grand prix or a football final.
★ Indulge yourself with a course of facials, manicures or massages.
★ Buy a pair of designer shoes.
★ Book a romantic weekend break or exotic holiday.

POTENTIAL PENALTIES
★ Not watching TV for a month.
★ Banning yourself from eating your favourite food for a month.
★ Postponing that haircut/root retouching you know you need.
★ Abstaining from alcohol for a month.
★ Volunteering to take your neighbour's horrid smelly dog for a walk every day for a month.
★ Doing all the grimmest household jobs like dehairing the shower plughole, taking out the rubbish or hoovering behind the sofa.

5 **Write it down** Along with this book, your daily diary (and your trainers!), your pen is your greatest ally in reaching your goal. Use it to complete the rest of your Mission Statement, to fill in the results of the fitness tests in Chapter Five and to schedule in each of The 60-Second-Secret Plan sessions (see Chapter Six) in your diary so you'll stick to your programme, stay focused and avoid getting side-tracked.

How's this for an amazing story that proves the power of the pen? In a study of students who'd recently graduated from Yale, only 3% said they'd written down specific goals for what they hoped to achieve in the future. Years later, when the graduates were surveyed again, the 3% who'd written down their goals had not only achieved most of what they'd hoped for, but their net worth equalled that of the other 97% combined. Worth trying for yourself, don't you think?

6 **Get going!** But not before you've done the four fabulous fitness tests in the next chapter. However, if you feel you really can't wait to get started, turn to page 66 to sneak a look at what the amazing 60-Second-Secret Plan has in store for you...

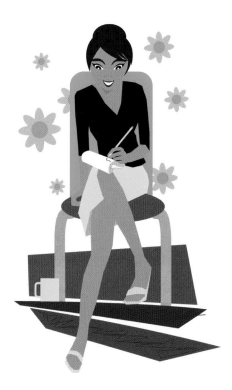

MY MISSION **STATEMENT**

I, _____**(name)**, being of sound mind, and slightly less sound body, do solemnly declare that I have decided to commit myself to getting fit. My **long-term dream goal** is to _____
_____,
which I aim to achieve by _____**(date)**. I have chosen this goal because (choose two of the **reasons** you ticked or wrote in your Why I Want To Get Fit list on page 43)

1._____
2._____
In order to achieve this long-term dream goal, I hereby commit myself to sticking faithfully to my short-term goals in The 60-Second-Secret Plan. I promise, every single time I complete a session from the plan, to **celebrate** by treating myself with a **Daily Reward** from the list on page 45. And at the end of every week that I've stuck to the programme, I'll celebrate by rewarding myself with
_____ (choose a **Weekly Treat** from the list on page 45). After successfully completing the programme, I'll celebrate by spoiling myself with _____
_____ (choose an **Ultimate Indulgence** from the list). I also promise faithfully to read this Mission Statement daily to remind myself of my goal (and my rewards!).
Today's date_____
Date I will have completed my short-term goals by (ten weeks' time)
_____
However, if I fail to complete The 60-Second-Secret Plan (odd lapses don't count!), I promise
to_____
(insert a penalty from the **Potential Penalties** list on page 45).

TOP TIP Photocopy this Mission Statement and keep a copy in your wallet, your daily diary or FiloFax and your gym bag. Stick a copy of it on your fridge door, next to your bathroom mirror or on your computer and look at it frequently to remind yourself of what you're determined to achieve. As Martin Luther King, Jr said, 'I have a dream…' Remember, you have one, too, now – all you have to do is go out and make it come true.

Here's why these people chose running as their goal
– and why they're still at it, and loving it, years later...

❝ Running's just awesome. Surfers have an expression, "Only a surfer knows the feeling," and it's the same with running. You can't describe it, you just have to feel it. **It's such a good feeling** when you're running tall and relaxed and your legs are just flowing through beneath you.'
Rob Banister, 24, facilities manager, Sydney, Australia

'In early 2002 I discovered **I had very high cholesterol levels and decided to change my diet radically**. As a result of eating more healthily and running, I've lost about 25.5kg (4st) and dropped from over 95.5kg (15st) to 70kg (11st), which is the weight I was when I started university. The more weight I lost, the more enjoyable running felt, until it became a pleasure in its own right. I'm amazed when I look back and realise that going for a run now at my old weight would be the equivalent of running with my six-year-old son sitting on my back!'
Duncan Edwards, 39, managing director, The National Magazine Company, London

'I have traumatic memories of cross-country races when all the other kids ran like aspiring athletes while I puffed along unhappily at the back, amazed that their lungs weren't on the verge of exploding from the lack of oxygen. Now that I'm running again 20 years later, I'm surprised it's so effortless – except, that is, when those dreaded hills loom and the emotions of a ten-year-old come flooding back into my 30-something being. I feel totally breathless, utterly hopeless and wretchedly miserable! And then I know why I run. It's because **it makes me feel young again!**'
Lize Lombard, lawyer, 32, Wimbledon

'**I run to keep fit and to relax**, and because I think a great deal when I'm running – I plan the day and wonder whom I'm going to drive crazy in the magazine business. During the week I live in London and follow the same running routine two or three times a week. I get up early and run a circuit that always passes the Houses of Parliament, where I check the time on Big Ben, before heading home again. Although as I get older I really have to discipline myself to do it, and sometimes it feels more like 30 miles than five or six, it makes me feel fresh, and sets me up for the day.'
Terry Mansfield CBE, 65, consultant, The Hearst Corporation, London

'I started running as part of a plan to get fitter, but now running is about more than just the exercise. **For me, it's about spending time alone**, outside, taking in the sights and sounds. Rather than punishing myself for stopping to catch my breath, I actually enjoy stopping to hear the birds or to admire a pretty front garden.' Sophie Easton, 33, crime scene examiner for the Metropolitan Police, Surrey

When you reach retirement, you can either choose to spend 20 years confined indoors watching endless reruns on the TV or **you can opt to pop out for a round of golf or perhaps a game of badminton with that nice person you've fancied for years!** The choice is yours. I know what I'd rather do – and that's why I run.' David Grant, 46, security officer, London

'On Saturday mornings I go running in the woods near my home. All I can hear is my breath and the crunching of snow. I'm constantly watching for moose that wander down from the hills when it gets cold. I'm a little more relaxed than when I run here in the summer, because the bears and their cubs are hibernating now. At about 10K (6 miles), I usually decide that it's time to head back. In the last few minutes of every run I do, **I take time to give thanks for the good things in my life** – the air in my lungs, the beauty I get to behold, the ability to love something such as running so much that my heart swells when I just think about it.'
Michael K Deems, Jr, 26, army officer, Fairbanks, Alaska, USA

'I run because even though I struggle with it, I know it's the absolute best thing I can do for my fitness. **I've never felt fitter than when I trained for a marathon.** Going for a bike ride or playing football just doesn't give you the same feeling. So I soldier on with it, even though I complain bitterly before every run!'
Adam Makepeace, 31, solicitor, London

'My wife always said she fell in love with me because **I had such good legs** – something I attribute to all the athletics I did at university. Reason enough, then, I thought, to carry on running once I left university. And so for 40 years I've gone for a 20-minute run after work each day. At 64, I'm proud to say I can still fit into the blazer I wore when I first met my wife!'
Anthony Jackson, 64, law student, Pretoria, South Africa

Are you ready to go on a voyage of self-discovery? Want to know the real you and what you're capable of? We've selected four key fitness tests and turned them into highly motivational tools you can use to track your progress and keep you inspired. Your first step to a fitter, more fabulous you starts right here...

5

get to know yourself

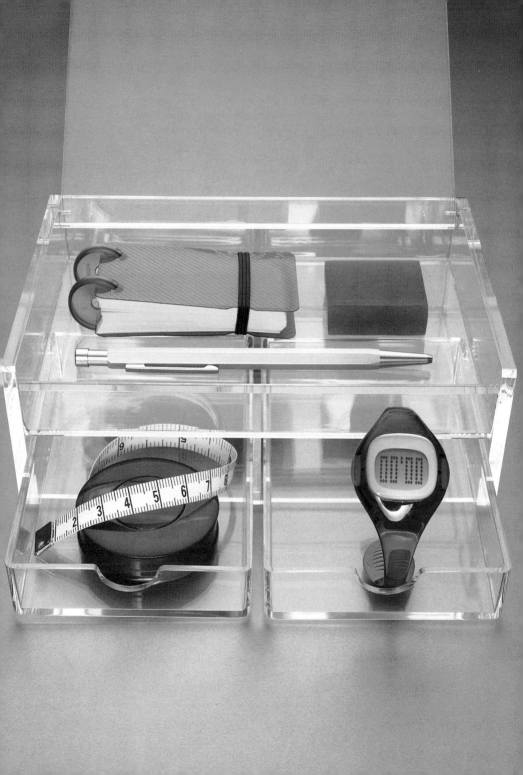

It's time to get cracking! You've completed your Mission Statement and now you need to establish how fit you are so you can monitor your progress as you shape up. Nothing will be more motivating than noting how your heartbeat slows as your fitness improves, watching those inches melt off, charting your weight loss as you gradually slim down and seeing your body-fat levels dropping.

Do I have to do all the tests?

No, but the more you do, the more you'll be able to bask in the glow of satisfaction that comes from knowing you're building a better, stronger, healthier body. Regularly doing these tests means you'll almost always have positive, concrete evidence of how much good your running programme is doing you.

The reason we've given you four to do is that even if you aren't quite as successful as you'd hoped in one area, such as weight loss, you'll still be able to see the real improvements you've made in other areas, such as your measurements. If you rely only on your scales to keep you motivated, you may be tempted to throw in the towel if there hasn't been any evidence of weight loss. However, if you also take your measurements, you'll notice that you've lost inches and can fit into your clothes more easily. Remember, changes in shape are just as important, healthwise, as weight loss. Reason enough to stick with the programme until you do lose some weight? You bet!

How should I do these tests?

To make sure these tests are as accurate as possible, do them at the same time of day (evening is best for monitoring your body-fat percentage, morning is best for the other three), wearing the same kind of clothing. Repeat them as directed to give you a clear idea of just how well you're doing. And don't forget to make a note in your diary to remind yourself to do them regularly.

Your self-test kit

✓ **Pen**
✓ **Pencil**
✓ **Tape measure**
✓ **Diary** (so you can note when you'll need to do the tests in the weeks and months to come)
✓ **Scales** (preferably those that can measure body-fat composition)
✓ **Watch** that can time seconds
✓ **Gym membership** or personal trainer (for body-fat percentage monitoring purposes – this is entirely optional!)

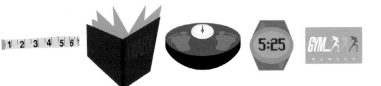

All about you: 4 fabulous fitness tests

TEST 1: RESTING HEART RATE

What you'll need

✓ Watch
✓ Pen

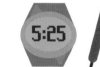

Why do it?

Measuring your heart rate (or pulse) when you're at rest is a good way to assess your cardiovascular fitness because the stronger your heart is, the fewer times a minute it has to pump to send blood around your body.

What to do

Do this test first thing in the morning so the results won't be affected by physical activities or stress. And avoid taking stimulants such as caffeine or nicotine before doing it.

Take your pulse at your wrist for 15 seconds, using your finger. Now multiply the number of heartbeats you counted by four to get your heart rate in beats per minute (bpm). If this figure is over 100, visit your GP as soon as you can as this may mean you have an abnormal heart rhythm that could potentially be dangerous.

What it all means

If you're running regularly, you can expect your resting heart rate to drop by one or two beats per minute every one to two weeks. If you've trained well, after six months you could be looking at a drop of between 10bpm and 15bpm. However, your heart rate will only drop a maximum of 20 beats.

MY RESTING HEART RATE

	Date / time	Resting heart rate in beats per minute
Today		
After 1 week		
After 2 weeks		
After 3 weeks		
After 4 weeks		
After 5 weeks		
After 6 weeks		
After 7 weeks		
After 8 weeks		
After 9 weeks		
After 10 weeks		
After 3 months		
After 4 months		
After 5 months		
After 6 months		

TEST 2: MEASUREMENTS

What you'll need

✓ **Tape measure**
✓ **Pen**

Why do it?

By measuring different parts of your body, you'll be able to keep track of how you're firming up and the way your body is changing as the fat melts away. Mind you, your declining bank balance as you regularly have to buy new clothes in smaller sizes will also be a brilliant indicator of how well you're doing!

Your waist measurement is probably the most important of the five measurements to focus on, as it can be a very valuable way to assess your health risks. This is because scientists now know that where you carry your extra weight can have a big impact on your health.

Pear-shaped people who have smaller waists and tend to carry extra weight on their hips and thighs are healthier than apple-shaped people who carry extra weight around their stomach. This is because fat comes in different types (yes, really!), and the type that is stored on the lower body is known as 'subcutaneous' and poses less of a health risk.

Fat that is stored deep within the abdomen, however, is known as 'visceral' and scientists now know it pumps out hormones and other substances that can lead to a range of health problems (see right).

What to do

Use the tape measure to take the measurements (in either inches or centimetres) of the following parts of your body – remember that for you to chart your progress accurately in the weeks and months to come, it's vital to take readings from the same place on each body part each time.

Chest: Place the tape measure around your chest so it runs across your nipples.

Waist: Place the tape measure around your waist so it runs straight across your tummy button.

Hips: Place the tape measure around your hips at the widest point.

Thigh: Place the tape measure around your leg at the highest part of your thigh, where it meets your groin.

Upper arm: Place the tape measure around your upper arm so it touches the highest part of your armpit.

What it all means

Again, your waist measurement is the key one. A waist that measures 80cm (31½in) or over in women and 94cm (37in) or over in men puts you at increased risk of type-2 diabetes.

If your waist measures over 89cm (35in) for a woman and over 102cm (40in) for a man, you're in the high-risk zone for type-2 diabetes and heart disease.

The other four measurements will help you track your weight-loss progress – and provide a constant source of motivation.

MY MEASUREMENTS

	Date	Chest	Waist	Hips	Thigh	Arm
Today						
After 1 week						
After 2 weeks						
After 3 weeks						
After 4 weeks						
After 5 weeks						
After 6 weeks						
After 7 weeks						
After 8 weeks						
After 9 weeks						
After 10 weeks						
After 3 months						
After 4 months						
After 5 months						
After 6 months						

TEST 3: WEIGHT AND BODY MASS INDEX (BMI)

What you'll need

✓ **Pencil**
✓ **Tape measure**
✓ **Pen**
✓ **Scales** (for consistency, always use the same set of scales)

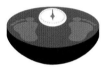

Why do it?

Your body mass index (BMI) expresses your weight in relation to your height and is used to work out whether you are overweight, underweight or just right for your height. It is sometimes criticised as not very accurate, because it doesn't directly take into account how much of your body weight is made up of fat and how much is made up of muscle. This means it can class very muscular but healthy people as overweight. However, for most of us, it's still a useful measurement, especially if you do it alongside the other tests that we recommend in this chapter.

What to do

1 Stand against a wall in your bare feet and, placing the pencil on top of your head, use it to draw a line lightly on the wall. Now measure the distance from the floor to the mark with the tape measure to get your height, and note it down in the My Weight & BMI chart (overleaf).

2 Next, strip down to your underwear (or your birthday suit, if you prefer), take a deep breath and hop on the scales. Now take another deep breath and open your eyes.

3 Allow yourself a secret smile if you like what you see, but if you don't, don't despair. Simply tell yourself, 'This is the heaviest I'm ever going to be, so there's no need to panic. I'll never be this weight again.'

4 Now make a note on the My Weight & BMI chart of your weight (in either kilograms or stones and pounds) and your weigh-in time and date, so that in future you can weigh yourself at more or less the same time of day.

5 Look at the Healthy Weight Range & BMI Table (right and overleaf) and calculate your BMI and healthy weight range – namely the area coloured green – and then fill in the rest of the chart overleaf.

6 Weigh yourself once a week and, for a really inspirational picture of your weight-loss progress, fill in the results on the graph on page 61. As your weight can fluctuate for a variety of reasons (such as how much you've just eaten or had to drink, whether you've just exercised, and so on), don't weigh yourself more than once a week, so your losses will have had time to accumulate.

HEALTHY WEIGHT RANGE & BMI TABLE

Height

BMI	15	16	17	18	19	20	21	22	23	24	25	26	27	28	29	30	31	32	33	34	35
1.47m 4ft 10in	32kg 5st 1lb	35kg 5st 7lb	37kg 5st 12lb	39kg 6st 2lb	41kg 6st 6lb	43kg 6st 11lb	45kg 7st 1lb	48kg 7st 8lb	50kg 7st 12lb	52kg 8st 3lb	54kg 8st 7lb	56kg 8st 11lb	58kg 9st 2lb	61kg 9st 8lb	63kg 9st 13lb	65kg 10st 3lb	67kg 10st 8lb	69kg 10st 12lb	71kg 11st 3lb	73kg 11st 7lb	76kg 12st
1.50m 4ft 11in	34kg 5st 5lb	36kg 5st 9lb	38kg 6st	41kg 6st 6lb	43kg 6st 11lb	45kg 7st 1lb	47kg 7st 6lb	50kg 7st 12lb	52kg 8st 3lb	54kg 8st 7lb	56kg 8st 11lb	59kg 9st 4lb	61kg 9st 8lb	63kg 9st 13lb	65kg 10st 3lb	68kg 10st 10lb	70kg 11st	72kg 11st 5lb	74kg 11st 9lb	77kg 12st 2lb	79kg 12st 6lb
1.52m 5ft	35kg 5st 7lb	37kg 5st 12lb	39kg 6st 2lb	42kg 6st 9lb	44kg 6st 13lb	46kg 7st 3lb	49kg 7st 10lb	51kg 8st	53kg 8st 5lb	55kg 8st 9lb	58kg 9st 2lb	60kg 9st 6lb	62kg 9st 11lb	65kg 10st 3lb	67kg 10st 8lb	69kg 10st 12lb	72kg 11st 5lb	74kg 11st 9lb	76kg 12st	79kg 12st 6lb	81kg 12st 11lb
1.55m 5ft 1in	36kg 5st 9lb	38kg 6st	41kg 6st 6lb	43kg 6st 11lb	46kg 7st 3lb	48kg 7st 8lb	50kg 7st 12lb	53kg 8st 5lb	55kg 8st 9lb	58kg 9st 2lb	60kg 9st 6lb	62kg 9st 11lb	65kg 10st 3lb	67kg 10st 8lb	70kg 11st	72kg 11st 5lb	74kg 11st 9lb	77kg 12st 2lb	79kg 12st 6lb	82kg 12st 13lb	84kg 13st 3lb
1.57m 5ft 2in	37kg 5st 12lb	39kg 6st 2lb	42kg 6st 9lb	44kg 6st 13lb	47kg 7st 6lb	49kg 7st 10lb	52kg 8st 3lb	54kg 8st 7lb	57kg 9st	59kg 9st 4lb	62kg 9st 11lb	64kg 10st 1lb	67kg 10st 8lb	69kg 10st 12lb	71kg 11st 3lb	74kg 11st 9lb	76kg 12st	79kg 12st 6lb	81kg 12st 11lb	84kg 13st 3lb	86kg 13st 8lb
1.6m 5ft 3in	38kg 6st	41kg 6st 6lb	44kg 6st 13lb	46kg 7st 3lb	49kg 7st 10lb	51kg 8st	54kg 8st 7lb	56kg 8st 11lb	59kg 9st 4lb	61kg 9st 8lb	64kg 10st 1lb	67kg 10st 8lb	69kg 10st 12lb	72kg 11st 5lb	74kg 11st 9lb	77kg 12st 2lb	79kg 12st 6lb	82kg 12st 13lb	84kg 13st 3lb	87kg 13st 10lb	90kg 14st 2lb
1.63m 5ft 4in	40kg 6st 4lb	43kg 6st 11lb	45kg 7st 1lb	48kg 7st 8lb	50kg 7st 12lb	53kg 8st 5lb	56kg 8st 11lb	58kg 9st 2lb	61kg 9st 8lb	64kg 10st 1lb	66kg 10st 6lb	69kg 10st 12lb	72kg 11st 5lb	74kg 11st 9lb	77kg 12st 2lb	80kg 12st 8lb	82kg 12st 13lb	85kg 13st 5lb	88kg 13st 12lb	90kg 14st 2lb	93kg 14st 9lb
1.65m 5ft 5in	41kg 6st 6lb	44kg 6st 13lb	46kg 7st 3lb	49kg 7st 10lb	52kg 8st 3lb	54kg 8st 7lb	57kg 9st	60kg 9st 6lb	63kg 9st 13lb	65kg 10st 3lb	68kg 10st 10lb	71kg 11st 3lb	74kg 11st 9lb	76kg 12st	79kg 12st 6lb	82kg 12st 13lb	84kg 13st 3lb	87kg 13st 10lb	90kg 14st 2lb	93kg 14st 9lb	95kg 14st 13lb
1.68m 5ft 6in	42kg 6st 9lb	45kg 7st 1lb	48kg 7st 8lb	51kg 8st	54kg 8st 7lb	56kg 8st 11lb	59kg 9st 4lb	62kg 9st 11lb	65kg 10st 3lb	68kg 10st 10lb	71kg 11st 3lb	73kg 11st 7lb	76kg 12st	79kg 12st 6lb	82kg 12st 13lb	85kg 13st 5lb	87kg 13st 10lb	90kg 14st 2lb	93kg 14st 9lb	96kg 15st 2lb	99kg 15st 8lb

Healthy weight range (BMI 20–25)

MY WEIGHT & BMI

My Height [ ]

My Healthy weight range [ ]

	Date/ weigh-in time	Weight	Weight loss	BMI	Dress size/ waist size
Today					
After 1 week					
After 2 weeks					
After 3 weeks					
After 4 weeks					
After 5 weeks					
After 6 weeks					
After 7 weeks					
After 8 weeks					
After 9 weeks					
After 10 weeks					
After 3 months					
After 4 months					
After 5 months					
After 6 months					

Height (BMI →)	15	16	17	18	19	20	21	22	23	24	25	26	27	28	29	30	31	32	33	34	35
1.7m 5ft 7in	44kg 6st 13lb	46kg 7st 3lb	49kg 7st 10lb	52kg 8st 3lb	55kg 8st 9lb	58kg 9st 2lb	61kg 9st 9lb	63kg 9st 13lb	67kg 10st 8lb	69kg 10st 12lb	72kg 11st 5lb	75kg 11st 11lb	78kg 12st 4lb	81kg 12st 11lb	84kg 13st 3lb	87kg 13st 10lb	90kg 14st 2lb	93kg 14st 9lb	96kg 15st 2lb	98kg 15st 6lb	101kg 15st 13lb
1.73m 5ft 8in	45kg 7st 1lb	48kg 7st 8lb	51kg 8st	54kg 8st 7lb	57kg 9st	60kg 9st 6lb	63kg 9st 13lb	66kg 10st 6lb	69kg 10st 12lb	72kg 11st 5lb	75kg 11st 11lb	78kg 12st 4lb	81kg 12st 11lb	84kg 13st 3lb	87kg 13st 10lb	90kg 14st 2lb	93kg 14st 9lb	96kg 15st 2lb	99kg 15st 8lb	102kg 16st 1lb	105kg 16st 8lb
1.75m 5ft 9in	46kg 7st 3lb	49kg 7st 10lb	52kg 8st 3lb	55kg 8st 9lb	58kg 9st 2lb	61kg 9st 9lb	64kg 10st 1lb	68kg 10st 10lb	71kg 11st 3lb	74kg 11st 9lb	76kg 12st	80kg 12st 8lb	83kg 13st 1lb	86kg 13st 8lb	89kg 14st	92kg 14st 7lb	95kg 14st 13lb	98kg 15st 6lb	101kg 15st 13lb	104kg 16st 5lb	107kg 16st 12lb
1.78m 5ft 10in	48kg 7st 8lb	51kg 8st	54kg 8st 7lb	57kg 9st	60kg 9st 6lb	63kg 9st 13lb	67kg 10st 8lb	70kg 11st	73kg 11st 7lb	76kg 12st	79kg 12st 6lb	82kg 12st 13lb	86kg 13st 8lb	89kg 14st	92kg 14st 7lb	95kg 14st 13lb	98kg 15st 6lb	101kg 15st 13lb	105kg 16st 8lb	108kg 17st	111kg 17st 7lb
1.8m 5ft 11in	49kg 7st 10lb	52kg 8st 3lb	55kg 8st 9lb	58kg 9st 2lb	62kg 9st 11lb	65kg 10st 3lb	68kg 10st 10lb	72kg 11st 5lb	75kg 11st 11lb	78kg 12st 4lb	81kg 12st 11lb	84kg 13st 3lb	87kg 13st 10lb	91kg 14st 5lb	94kg 14st 11lb	98kg 15st 6lb	101kg 15st 13lb	104kg 16st 5lb	107kg 16st 12lb	110kg 17st 5lb	113kg 17st 11lb
1.83m 6ft	50kg 7st 12lb	54kg 8st 7lb	57kg 9st	60kg 9st 6lb	63kg 9st 13lb	67kg 10st 8lb	70kg 11st	73kg 11st 7lb	77kg 12st 2lb	80kg 12st 8lb	83kg 13st 1lb	87kg 13st 10lb	90kg 14st 2lb	94kg 14st 11lb	97kg 15st 4lb	100kg 15st 10lb	104kg 16st 5lb	107kg 16st 12lb	111kg 17st 7lb	114kg 17st 13lb	117kg 18st 6lb
1.85m 6ft 1in	51kg 8st	55kg 8st 9lb	59kg 9st 4lb	62kg 9st 11lb	65kg 10st 3lb	69kg 10st 12lb	72kg 11st 5lb	76kg 12st	79kg 12st 6lb	82kg 12st 13lb	86kg 13st 8lb	89kg 14st	93kg 14st 9lb	96kg 15st 2lb	100kg 15st 10lb	103kg 16st 3lb	106kg 16st 10lb	110kg 17st 5lb	113kg 17st 11lb	117kg 18st 6lb	120kg 18st 13lb
1.88m 6ft 2in	53kg 8st 5lb	57kg 9st	60kg 9st 6lb	64kg 10st 1lb	67kg 10st 8lb	71kg 11st 3lb	74kg 11st 9lb	78kg 12st 4lb	81kg 12st 11lb	84kg 13st 3lb	88kg 13st 12lb	92kg 14st 7lb	95kg 14st 13lb	99kg 15st 8lb	103kg 16st 3lb	106kg 16st 10lb	110kg 17st 5lb	113kg 17st 11lb	117kg 18st 6lb	120kg 18st 13lb	124kg 19st 7lb
1.9m 6ft 3in	54kg 8st 7lb	58kg 9st 2lb	62kg 9st 11lb	65kg 10st 3lb	69kg 10st 12lb	73kg 11st 7lb	76kg 12st	80kg 12st 8lb	83kg 13st 1lb	87kg 13st 10lb	91kg 14st 5lb	94kg 14st 11lb	98kg 15st 6lb	101kg 15st 13lb	105kg 16st 8lb	109kg 17st 2lb	112kg 17st 9lb	116kg 18st 4lb	120kg 18st 13lb	123kg 19st 6lb	126kg 19st 12lb
1.93m 6ft 4in	56kg 8st 12lb	60kg 9st 6lb	63kg 9st 13lb	67kg 10st 8lb	71kg 11st 3lb	74kg 11st 9lb	78kg 12st 4lb	82kg 12st 13lb	86kg 13st 8lb	89kg 14st	93kg 14st 9lb	97kg 15st 4lb	101kg 15st 13lb	104kg 16st 5lb	107kg 16st 12lb	112kg 17st 9lb	116kg 18st 4lb	119kg 18st 10lb	123kg 19st 6lb	127kg 20st	130kg 20st 6lb

Healthy weight range (BMI 19–24)

Height

Adapted from a BMI chart supplied courtesy of Weight Watchers (www.weightwatchers.co.uk)

What it all means

BMI below 18.5 — You are underweight and should get medical advice before starting a running programme as it could make your weight drop even further. Being severely underweight is more of a problem for women than men as it may mean you stop having periods, which can increase your risk of osteoporosis.

BMI of 18.5 – 24.9 — You are within the ideal weight range for your height – good for you! Taking up running will help you keep up the good work.

BMI of 25 – 29.9 — You are on the tubby side – running will help you gradually move towards a healthier weight.

BMI of 30+ — You are seriously overweight and so should improve your diet and start doing regular exercise (and, you'll burn even more calories – and get more bang for your buck! – if you combine running with weight-training). Don't forget to see your GP before you start, though.

For added motivation, colour in this graph (right) once a week to get a visual picture of the difference that running is making to your weight. Each block represents 1kg or 2lb (remember always to use the same unit of measurement). And don't forget to draw two thick lines across the graph to show your healthy weight range (see the Healthy Weight Range & BMI Table on pages 57 and 59), which will give you something to aim for.

MY WEIGHT-LOSS GRAPH

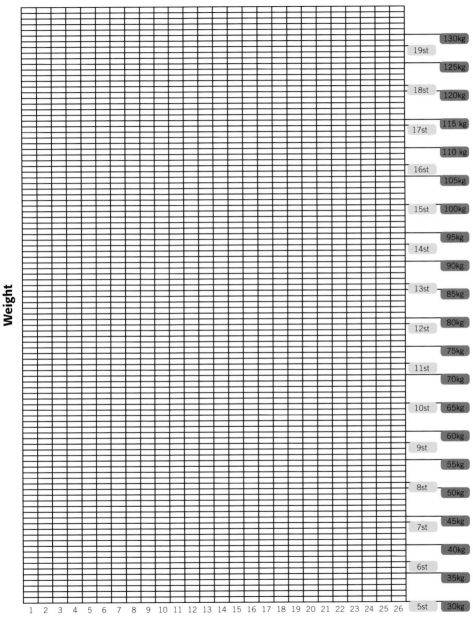

Weeks

Each block = 1kg or 2lb

TEST 4: BODY-FAT PERCENTAGE

What you'll need

✓ **Pen**
✓ **Scales with a body-fat monitor function** (for consistency, always use the same ones)
   OR
✓ **Gym membership or access to a personal trainer**

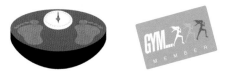

This test measures the percentage of fat in your body. It's the only one of the four tests that requires specialist equipment (or a personal trainer or gym membership), which can be a bit pricey, so don't worry if you can't manage to do it. However, remember that being able to see that your body fat is burning off and your muscle tissue is increasing is highly motivating and will give you a more accurate picture of your health.

Why do it?

Simply measuring your weight alone isn't a clear indicator of good health because ordinary scales aren't psychic – they can't tell the difference between weight that comes from fat and weight that comes from lean body tissue (muscles, bones, organs and blood). This means it's possible for your weight to be in the ideal range yet your body-fat level to be on the high side. Why is it important to be aware of how much body fat you have? Well,

if your level is excessively high, you're at risk of getting some very nasty diseases such as heart disease, arthritis, type-2 diabetes and some types of cancer, and the risk soars as your body-fat level increases. If your body fat is excessively low, this can lead to increased risk of osteoporosis, a decrease in fertility and even amenorrhoea, a condition in which women cease to have periods.

Something else to bear in mind is that 450g (1lb) of fat tissue burns only two calories in 24 hours, whereas 450g (1lb) of muscle burns about 35 calories, so the more muscle you have, the more calories you'll burn. Adding just a little muscle makes a big difference to the number of calories you use a day. A kilogram (2lb) of muscle burns an extra 70 calories a day – that's 2,100 calories per month, equivalent to losing 225g (more than half a pound) of fat. And that's *without* changing your diet!

Monitoring your body fat is really helpful if you're trying to lose weight and don't seem to be getting anywhere (been there, done that?) because it will prove to you that your workout plan is actually working. It'll show you that you're replacing fat with muscle, which, because it's heavier than fat, can make you despair at having gained weight.

How is it done?

Body fat can be measured in a variety of ways. One method involves using a body-fat monitor, which works on the principle of bio-electrical impedance (BIA). It sounds scary, but what this means is that a very low, safe, painless electrical signal is passed through your body (however, it shouldn't be used by pregnant women or those with pacemakers). This signal whizzes through the fluids in lean tissue but has difficulty getting through fat tissue. The body-fat monitor measures this difficulty (hence the term bio-electrical *impedance*) and then uses the additional information you've given it, such as your sex and height, to calculate your body-fat percentage.

The good news is that body-fat monitors aren't available solely to gymgoers and athletes – you can use one in the privacy of your own home. Tanita makes the best-known brand of monitor, which handily doubles up as conventional scales (29% of Japanese people own one!). Another reputable but less well-known brand is Salter. (For stockists, visit www.tanita.com and www.salterhousewares.com.)

What to do

If you have scales that double as a body-fat monitor, programme them according to the instructions and take your reading. Always do the test at the same time of day so you're comparing like with like. The best time to do this test is in the early evening, before a meal, when you're more likely to be fully hydrated. Follow the manufacturer's instructions to the letter, as things such as not going to the loo before the test or when you last ate or drank can distort your results. This is because these things can raise or lower the amount of water in your body, which affects the amount of resistance it'll put up to the electrical signal. Alternatively, ask an instructor at your gym (or a personal trainer) to do the test for you.

MY BODY-FAT PERCENTAGE

	Date/ time	Body-fat percentage
Today		
After 1 week		
After 2 weeks		
After 3 weeks		
After 4 weeks		
After 5 weeks		
After 6 weeks		
After 7 weeks		
After 8 weeks		
After 9 weeks		
After 10 weeks		
After 3 months		
After 4 months		
After 5 months		
After 6 months		

What it all means
This chart will give you an indication of the healthy ranges to aim for:

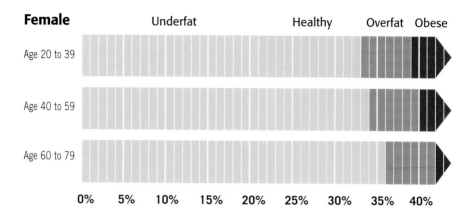

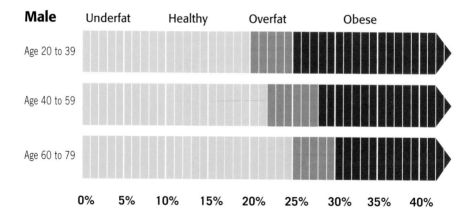

National Institutes of Health/World Health Organisation BMI guidelines, as reported by Gallagher at the New York Obesity Research Center, based on data from the *American Journal of Clinical Nutrition* 2000; 72: 694-701. Data used with permission of the *American Journal of Clinical Nutrition* © Am J Clin Nutr American Society For Clinical Nutrition

And finally...

Once you've done all the tests, fill in your scores on the How I Measure Up Today chart (below), then after six months' worth of exercise and tests, fill in the How I Measure Up In Six Months' Time chart (below) to see exactly how much progress you've made. We guarantee you'll be amazed!

HOW I MEASURE UP TODAY

Today's date _____

Dress/clothing size _____

Weight _____

BMI _____

Body-fat percentage _____
Body measurements

Chest _____

Waist _____

Hips _____

Thigh _____

Arm _____

Resting heart rate _____

HOW I MEASURE UP IN SIX MONTHS' TIME

Date _____

Dress/clothing size _____

Weight _____

BMI _____

Body-fat percentage _____
Body measurements

Chest _____

Waist _____

Hips _____

Thigh _____

Arm _____

Resting heart rate _____

Here's the moment you've been waiting for – you're about to meet your perfect running plan and take your first steps towards a new, improved you…

6

get going

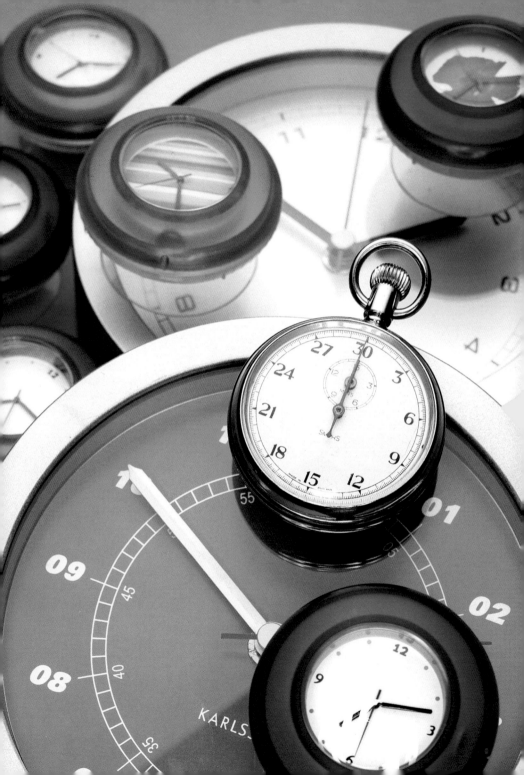

Feeling inspired? Raring to have a go at running? Then it's time to hop off that sofa, lace up your trainers and start our ultra-easy 60-Second-Secret Plan…

We invented The 60-Second-Secret Plan because everyone, no matter how unfit or unconfident, can manage to run for 60 seconds. What counts isn't how fast you go or how far you get in one minute. In fact, quite the opposite – the idea is to go slow and steady (doing anything from a barely-more-than-walking shuffle to a steady jog), take a walk break to get your breath back, then do it again. What we really don't want you to do is make the classic beginner's mistake and go hurtling out of your front door only to burn out in seconds.

And along with rubbishing the idea that the only way to run is fast, we also want you to stop thinking of taking walk breaks as wrong. Walking during your runs isn't an admission of defeat but a smart way to improve. 'Walk breaks are a vital part of the programme because, if you've never run before, it's crucial to take things really slowly so your body gets the time it needs to adapt to the new things you're asking it to do,' says Kirsty O'Neill, who leads Cannons/Reebok walk-to-run clubs in Northampton, and helped devise The 60-Second-Secret Plan. 'Taking walk breaks means you can keep going for longer without getting too tired.' Walk breaks also

mean you're getting a more complete workout because you're using lots of different muscles, and you're also reducing your risk of injury.

The 60-Second-Secret Plan doesn't just make physical sense, it's also designed to work where other plans have failed because it's so motivating, empowering and fun. Plus, because it's broken down into easy-to-manage 60-second chunks, you'll always feel more than capable of doing what's asked of you. 'I've found from leading walk-to-run groups over the years that for people to achieve something, they first have to believe they're able to do it,' says O'Neill. 'That's why having an easy goal such as running for just 60 seconds is at the core of the plan – it's something everyone feels they can do.' Even if you're already a proficient runner, The 60-Second-Secret Plan can still help you. 'When I started a walk-run plan, I could already run for 30 minutes,' says Bonnie Jarvis, a vet from Tucson, USA. 'However, my trainer insisted it would improve my running. Now I can run for an hour and still feel great.'

Can't wait to start? Here are just a few things you need to do first…

Gear up!

The only gear you need to get started is a good pair of trainers and – if you're a woman – a sports bra. Swanky T-shirts and sweatpants can come later on, but don't skimp on your trainers and bra as you want to stay comfortable and, above all, injury-free. (There's a complete lowdown on the best trainers and sports bras to buy in Chapter Seven.) Oh, and you'll also need a really simple digital watch or stopwatch that records seconds, so you can measure how long to run or walk for.

Drink up!

Fill a water bottle and make sure you sip water before, during and after your sessions as staying hydrated when exercising is vital (for more on this, see tip 4 in Chapter Seven).

Write up!

At the start of every week, find a time slot for each of the four sessions (before or after work, during your lunch hour, whenever) and mark them in your daily diary to help you stick 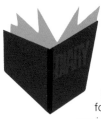 to them. Don't forget, either, to fill in the time your session is planned for and the rewards you're promising yourself for completing each one in the Fill-It-In 60-Second-Secret Plan, which starts on page 73.

Each session in the plan also has a Mood-O-Meter so you can monitor how you feel before, during and after your run, and you can see at a glance just how much good your running is doing you mentally.

Warm up!

Begin each session with 5 minutes of brisk walking to prepare your body, then do the four gentle stretches on pages 116 and 117. After your session, walk slowly for 5 minutes to cool down, then stretch again (see page 118). Instead of seeing your stretches as a chore, think of the time you spend doing them as an oasis of calm in a busy day or a chance to reflect on just how well you've done in completing the session.

Steady up!

And finally, remember, DO NOT RACE! The idea is to start out very slow and steady and complete the session, rather than burn out in ten seconds and vow you'll never go running again. When we say 'run' we mean find a pace that's faster than a walk – waddling, shuffling, staggering, jogging or really stepping it out all count.

If you're already fit, you might manage a good running pace. But remember, there's no right or wrong here – just like driving, you can run in any gear! What counts is that you feel as if you're working and challenging yourself a little, but not killing yourself and gasping for breath. When you take your walk break, the idea is to slow down enough to recover, but try to stay at a brisk rather than at a window-shopping pace!

YOUR AT-A-GLANCE 60-SECOND-SECRET PLAN

Photocopy this plan and keep it with you if you don't want to carry *Running Made Easy* everywhere. See overleaf for a longer, more interactive version of this plan. (The times in brackets are the totals for each of your sessions.)

WEEK ONE
Monday: Run 60 secs, walk 3 mins. Repeat 3 more times (16 mins)
Tuesday: Rest
Wednesday: Run 60 secs, walk 3 mins. Repeat 3 more times (16 mins)
Thursday: Rest
Friday: Run 60 secs, walk 3 mins. Repeat 3 more times (16 mins)
Saturday: Rest
Sunday: 30-minute brisk walk

WEEK TWO
Monday: Run 60 secs, walk 2 mins. Repeat 5 more times (18 mins)
Tuesday: Rest
Wednesday: Run 60 secs, walk 2 mins. Repeat 5 more times (18 mins)
Thursday: Rest
Friday: Run 60 secs, walk 2 mins. Repeat 5 more times (18 mins)
Saturday: Rest
Sunday: 30-minute brisk walk

WEEK THREE
Monday: Run 60 secs, walk 2 mins. Repeat 6 more times (21 mins)
Tuesday: Rest
Wednesday: Run 60 secs, walk 2 mins. Repeat 6 more times (21 mins)
Thursday: Rest
Friday: Run 60 secs, walk 2 mins. Repeat 6 more times (21 mins)
Saturday: Rest
Sunday: 30-minute brisk walk

WEEK FOUR
Monday: Run 60 secs, walk 2 mins. Repeat 7 more times (24 mins)
Tuesday: Rest
Wednesday: Run 60 secs, walk 2 mins. Repeat 7 more times (24 mins)
Thursday: Rest
Friday: Run 60 secs, walk 2 mins. Repeat 7 more times (24 mins)
Saturday: Rest
Sunday: 35-minute brisk walk

WEEK FIVE
Monday: Run 60 secs, walk 2 mins. Repeat 8 more times (27 mins)
Tuesday: Rest
Wednesday: Do a different kind of exercise session – anything from brisk walking, swimming or cycling to weights or an aerobics class. Aim for a 30-minute gentle workout or a mix of two 15-minute workouts adding up to 30 minutes
Thursday: Rest
Friday: Run 60 secs, walk 2 mins. Repeat 8 more times (27 mins)
Saturday: Rest
Sunday: Run 60 secs, walk 2 mins. Repeat 8 more times (27 mins)

WEEK SIX
Monday: Run 2 mins, walk 2 mins. Repeat 6 more times (28 mins)
Tuesday: Rest
Wednesday: Free session – 30 minutes' brisk walking/dancing/ cycling/ swimming/weights – whatever you like!
Thursday: Rest
Friday: Run 2 mins, walk 2 mins. Repeat 6 more times (28 mins)
Saturday: Rest
Sunday: Run 2 mins, walk 2 mins. Repeat 6 more times (28 mins)

WEEK SEVEN
Monday: Run 2 mins, walk 2 mins. Repeat 7 more times (32 mins)
Tuesday: Rest
Wednesday: Free session – 30 minutes to do a fun activity!
Thursday: Rest
Friday: Run 2 mins, walk 2 mins. Repeat 7 more times (32 mins)
Saturday: Rest
Sunday: Run 2 mins, walk 2 mins. Repeat 7 more times (32 mins)

WEEK EIGHT
Monday: Run 3 mins, walk 2 mins. Repeat 6 more times (35 mins)
Tuesday: Rest
Wednesday: Try to increase your free session to 40 minutes
Thursday: Rest
Friday: Run 3 mins, walk 2 mins. Repeat 6 more times (35 mins)
Saturday: Rest
Sunday: Run 3 mins, walk 2 mins. Repeat 6 more times (35 mins)

WEEK NINE
Monday: Run 3 mins, walk 2 mins. Repeat 6 more times (35 mins)
Tuesday: Rest
Wednesday: Free session – 40 minutes of any activity you choose – and don't forget to have fun!
Thursday: Rest
Friday: Run 3 mins, walk 60 secs. Repeat 8 more times (36 mins)
Saturday: Rest
Sunday: Run 3 mins, walk 60 secs. Repeat 8 more times (36 mins)

WEEK TEN
Monday: Run 3 mins, walk 60 secs. Repeat 8 more times (36 mins)
Tuesday: Rest
Wednesday: 40-minute free session
Thursday: Rest
Friday: Run 3 mins, walk 60 secs. Repeat 8 more times (36 mins)
Saturday: Rest
Sunday: Run 3 mins, walk 60 secs. Repeat 9 more times (40 mins)

CONGRATULATIONS!
You're now capable of running/walking for 40 minutes, which should easily get you around a 5K (3-mile) race. If you're feeling good on the final Sunday session and want to push yourself a little more, you can simply keep running for as long as you're able to, then slow down for a walk break when you need one, and repeat until you've gone for 40 minutes. For example, you might run for 9 minutes, walk for 1 minute, and then repeat four times.

YOUR FILL-IT-IN 60-SECOND-SECRET PLAN
(complete with Mood-O-Meter)

Use our unique Mood-O-Meter to measure your mood before, during and after every run and you'll soon realise that even on those days when running feels like the very last thing you want to do, you'll absolutely always feel like a million dollars afterwards. Read on to discover what the Mood-O-Meter's cute little symbols (below) really mean...

HOW YOU FELT... BEFORE YOUR RUN

 HELLISH Wild horses had to drag me out of the door. I did not want to run today.

 INDIFFERENT I went out because I was scheduled to, not because I wanted to.

 UP AND DOWN I was in two minds whether to go running or not.

 GOOD I had no problem getting going today – I felt fit and positive.

 EUPHORIC I was itching to go out for a run – nothing could hold me back.

HOW YOU FELT... DURING YOUR RUN

 HELLISH That was simply awful! I loathed every second. My breath came in ragged gasps and I had logs for legs.

 INDIFFERENT That was the equivalent of a school dinner – dull and uneventful.

 UP AND DOWN There were bad bits, but good bits, too. As soon as I got going, I felt better.

 GOOD I enjoyed my run – my legs felt strong and I felt in control the whole time.

 EUPHORIC Running? I was flying! Hill? What hill? I could have gone on for ever – and then some.

HOW YOU FELT... AFTER YOUR RUN

 HELLISH Eugh! I really hated that and felt terrible afterwards.

 INDIFFERENT Errrr, that was a bit grim. But it was bearable... I guess.

 UP AND DOWN Hmmm, I loved and hated it in equal measure.

 GOOD I felt great – relaxed, invigorated and extremely proud of myself.

 EUPHORIC Wow! I felt elated and couldn't wait to go and do it all over again.

Week One

> **66** The miracle isn't that I finished – the miracle is that I had the courage to start **99**
> John Bingham, motivational expert

MONDAY Run 60 secs, walk 3 mins. Repeat 3 more times (Total: 16 mins)
Time of day you're planning to run:_____
Mood before: ☹ ☺ ☺ ☺ ☺ Mood during: ☹ ☺ ☺ ☺ ☺ Mood after: ☹ ☺ ☺ ☺ ☺
Daily Reward _____

TUESDAY Rest

WEDNESDAY Run 60 secs, walk 3 mins. Repeat 3 more times (Total: 16 mins)
Time of day you're planning to run:_____
Mood before: ☹ ☺ ☺ ☺ ☺ Mood during: ☹ ☺ ☺ ☺ ☺ Mood after: ☹ ☺ ☺ ☺ ☺
Daily Reward _____

THURSDAY Rest

FRIDAY Run 60 secs, walk 3 mins. Repeat 3 more times (Total: 16 mins)
Time of day you're planning to run:_____
Mood before: ☹ ☺ ☺ ☺ ☺ Mood during: ☹ ☺ ☺ ☺ ☺ Mood after: ☹ ☺ ☺ ☺ ☺
Daily Reward _____

SATURDAY Rest

SUNDAY 30-minute brisk walk
Time of day you're planning to walk:_____
Mood before: ☹ ☺ ☺ ☺ ☺ Mood during: ☹ ☺ ☺ ☺ ☺ Mood after: ☹ ☺ ☺ ☺ ☺
Weekly Treat _____

You may be feeling... weak and wobbly. You may feel like Bambi on ice (both during and after your session!), and your bottom may feel as if it's jiggling around like jelly on a plate, but don't let this put you off. It's only a temporary phase as running is one of the fastest ways on the planet to get fit and firm up. Even really experienced runners feel bad after a long lay-off. It really doesn't matter what you look or feel like right now the important thing, as the quote above says, is that you've had the courage to start.

Week Two

❝It is the greatest of all mistakes to do nothing because you can only do a little. Do what you can ❞
Sydney Smith, essayist

MONDAY Run 60 secs, walk 2 mins. Repeat 5 more times (Total: 18 mins)
Time of day you're planning to run:_____
Mood before: ☹ ☹ ☺ ☺ ☺ Mood during: ☹ ☹ ☺ ☺ ☺ Mood after: ☹ ☹ ☺ ☺ ☺
Daily Reward _____

TUESDAY Rest

WEDNESDAY Run 60 secs, walk 2 mins. Repeat 5 more times (Total: 18 mins)
Time of day you're planning to run:_____
Mood before: ☹ ☹ ☺ ☺ ☺ Mood during: ☹ ☹ ☺ ☺ ☺ Mood after: ☹ ☹ ☺ ☺ ☺
Daily Reward _____

THURSDAY Rest

FRIDAY Run 60 secs, walk 2 mins. Repeat 5 more times (Total: 18 mins)
Time of day you're planning to run:_____
Mood before: ☹ ☹ ☺ ☺ ☺ Mood during: ☹ ☹ ☺ ☺ ☺ Mood after: ☹ ☹ ☺ ☺ ☺
Daily Reward _____

SATURDAY Rest

SUNDAY 30-minute brisk walk
Time of day you're planning to walk:_____
Mood before: ☹ ☹ ☺ ☺ ☺ Mood during: ☹ ☹ ☺ ☺ ☺ Mood after: ☹ ☹ ☺ ☺ ☺
Weekly Treat _____

You may be feeling... puffed out. But this is perfectly normal – you'll need to breathe a bit faster because your body needs more oxygen to fuel its efforts. (As you get fitter, you'll definitely feel less breathless.) However, you shouldn't be gasping for breath – if you're practically hyperventilating, just slow down and do what you can. A simple way to make sure you're not overdoing it is to take the Talk Test. If you can talk, you're running at the right pace, but if you can sing, you're not making enough effort.

66 All good things are difficult to achieve; and bad things are very easy to get 99
Morarji Desai, former Indian prime minister

MONDAY Run 60 secs, walk 2 mins. Repeat 6 more times (Total: 21 mins)
Time of day you're planning to run:_____
Mood before: 😝 😐 😕 😊 😃 Mood during: 😝 😐 😕 😊 😃 Mood after: 😝 😐 😕 😊 😃
Daily Reward _____

TUESDAY Rest

WEDNESDAY Run 60 secs, walk 2 mins. Repeat 6 more times (Total: 21 mins)
Time of day you're planning to run:_____
Mood before: 😝 😐 😕 😊 😃 Mood during: 😝 😐 😕 😊 😃 Mood after: 😝 😐 😕 😊 😃
Daily Reward _____

THURSDAY Rest

FRIDAY Run 60 secs, walk 2 mins. Repeat 6 more times (Total: 21 mins)
Time of day you're planning to run:_____
Mood before: 😝 😐 😕 😊 😃 Mood during: 😝 😐 😕 😊 😃 Mood after: 😝 😐 😕 😊 😃
Daily Reward _____

SATURDAY Rest

SUNDAY 30-minute brisk walk
Time of day you're planning to walk:_____
Mood before: 😝 😐 😕 😊 😃 Mood during: 😝 😐 😕 😊 😃 Mood after: 😝 😐 😕 😊 😃
Weekly Treat _____

You may be feeling… stiff and sore. Muscles that you never knew you had will come kicking and screaming to the surface and demand your attention. Make sure you help your body to adapt by always stretching properly after every run (see tip 54 in Chapter Seven), and try soaking in a warm bath to get rid of aches and pains. And if you have some spare cash, treat yourself to a massage to help soothe sore muscles and get you feeling blissfully relaxed.

Week Four

66 Take the first step in faith. You don't have to see the whole staircase, just take the first step 99
Martin Luther King, Jr, civil rights leader

MONDAY Run 60 secs, walk 2 mins. Repeat 7 more times (Total: 24 mins)
Time of day you're planning to run:_____
Mood before: ☹😐😕🙂😊 Mood during: ☹😐😕🙂😊 Mood after: ☹😐😕🙂😊
Daily Reward _____

TUESDAY Rest

WEDNESDAY Run 60 secs, walk 2 mins. Repeat 7 more times (Total: 24 mins)
Time of day you're planning to run:_____
Mood before: ☹😐😕🙂😊 Mood during: ☹😐😕🙂😊 Mood after: ☹😐😕🙂😊
Daily Reward _____

THURSDAY Rest

FRIDAY Run 60 secs, walk 2 mins. Repeat 7 more times (Total: 24 mins)
Time of day you're planning to run:_____
Mood before: ☹😐😕🙂😊 Mood during: ☹😐😕🙂😊 Mood after: ☹😐😕🙂😊
Daily Reward _____

SATURDAY Rest

SUNDAY 35-minute brisk walk
Time of day you're planning to walk:_____
Mood before: ☹😐😕🙂😊 Mood during: ☹😐😕🙂😊 Mood after: ☹😐😕🙂😊
Weekly Treat _____

You may be feeling... unsure if you're really doing it right,
if it's ever going to work – or even if you want to continue doing it at all.
Don't worry, everyone has beginner's doubts. Stick at it – your confidence,
like your fitness, will grow every time you finish a session until running starts
feeling like the most natural thing in the world.

❝ This is no time for ease and comfort. It is time to dare and endure ❞
Winston Churchill, former British prime minister

MONDAY Run 60 secs, walk 2 mins. Repeat 8 more times (Total: 27 mins)
Time of day you're planning to run:_____
Mood before: ☹ ☹ 😐 ☺ 😄 Mood during: ☹ ☹ 😐 ☺ 😄 Mood after: ☹ ☹ 😐 ☺ 😄
Daily Reward _____

TUESDAY Rest

WEDNESDAY Swap in a different kind of exercise session here – do anything
from brisk walking, swimming or cycling to weights or an aerobics class.
Aim for a 30-minute gentle workout – doing either just one activity or a mix
of two 15-minute or three 10-minute workouts adding up to 30 minutes
Time of day you're planning to exercise:_____
Mood before: ☹ ☹ 😐 ☺ 😄 Mood during: ☹ ☹ 😐 ☺ 😄 Mood after: ☹ ☹ 😐 ☺ 😄
Daily Reward _____

THURSDAY Rest

FRIDAY Run 60 secs, walk 2 mins. Repeat 8 more times (Total: 27 mins)
Time of day you're planning to run:_____
Mood before: ☹ ☹ 😐 ☺ 😄 Mood during: ☹ ☹ 😐 ☺ 😄 Mood after: ☹ ☹ 😐 ☺ 😄
Daily Reward _____

SATURDAY Rest

SUNDAY Run 60 secs, walk 2 mins. Repeat 8 more times (Total: 27 mins)
Time of day you're planning to run:_____
Mood before: ☹ ☹ 😐 ☺ 😄 Mood during: ☹ ☹ 😐 ☺ 😄 Mood after: ☹ ☹ 😐 ☺ 😄
Weekly Treat _____

You may be feeling... like giving up. Don't! You've come halfway and
it'll all get easier from now on. When you're feeling weak-willed, think back
to how much effort you've made and what a shame it would be to waste it.
Think about how far you've already come – admit it, just a few weeks ago the
thought of exercising for 30 minutes was enough to turn your stomach!

Week Six

> ❝ Sweat cleanses from the inside. It comes from places a shower will never reach ❞
>
> George Sheehan, writer

MONDAY Run 2 mins, walk 2 mins. Repeat 6 more times (Total: 28 mins)
Time of day you're planning to run:_____
Mood before: ☹ ☹ ☺ ☺ ☺ Mood during: ☹ ☹ ☺ ☺ ☺ Mood after: ☹ ☹ ☺ ☺ ☺
Daily Reward _____

TUESDAY Rest

WEDNESDAY Free session – 30 minutes' brisk walking/dancing/cycling/
swimming/weights – whatever you like!
Time of day you're planning to exercise:_____
Mood before: ☹ ☹ ☺ ☺ ☺ Mood during: ☹ ☹ ☺ ☺ ☺ Mood after: ☹ ☹ ☺ ☺ ☺
Daily Reward _____

THURSDAY Rest

FRIDAY Run 2 mins, walk 2 mins. Repeat 6 more times (Total: 28 mins)
Time of day you're planning to run:_____
Mood before: ☹ ☹ ☺ ☺ ☺ Mood during: ☹ ☹ ☺ ☺ ☺ Mood after: ☹ ☹ ☺ ☺ ☺
Daily Reward _____

SATURDAY Rest

SUNDAY Run 2 mins, walk 2 mins. Repeat 6 more times (Total: 28 mins)
Time of day you're planning to run:_____
Mood before: ☹ ☹ ☺ ☺ ☺ Mood during: ☹ ☹ ☺ ☺ ☺ Mood after: ☹ ☹ ☺ ☺ ☺
Weekly Treat _____

You may be feeling... sweaty, especially as you're now having to get used to running for 2 minutes at a stretch. But don't be grossed out by your own sweat – see it rather as a badge of courage, something you've earned. Remember that you can lose up to 500ml/1 pint of sweat per 30-minute workout, so drink plenty of water before, during and after your sessions. Experts recommend that you drink between half a teacup to a teacup every ten to 20 minutes when you're exercising.

66 I've got my faults, but living in the past isn't one of them. There's no future in it 99
Sparky Anderson, baseball coach

MONDAY Run 2 mins, walk 2 mins. Repeat 7 more times (Total: 32 mins)
Time of day you're planning to run:_____
Mood before: ☹ ☺ ☺ ☺ ☺ Mood during: ☹ ☺ ☺ ☺ ☺ Mood after: ☹ ☺ ☺ ☺ ☺
Daily Reward _____

TUESDAY Rest

WEDNESDAY Free session – 30 minutes to do a fun activity!
Time of day you're planning to exercise:_____
Mood before: ☹ ☺ ☺ ☺ ☺ Mood during: ☹ ☺ ☺ ☺ ☺ Mood after: ☹ ☺ ☺ ☺ ☺
Daily Reward _____

THURSDAY Rest

FRIDAY Run 2 mins, walk 2 mins. Repeat 7 more times (Total: 32 mins)
Time of day you're planning to run:_____
Mood before: ☹ ☺ ☺ ☺ ☺ Mood during: ☹ ☺ ☺ ☺ ☺ Mood after: ☹ ☺ ☺ ☺ ☺
Daily Reward _____

SATURDAY Rest

SUNDAY Run 2 mins, walk 2 mins. Repeat 7 more times (Total: 32 mins)
Time of day you're planning to run:_____
Mood before: ☹ ☺ ☺ ☺ ☺ Mood during: ☹ ☺ ☺ ☺ ☺ Mood after: ☹ ☺ ☺ ☺ ☺
Weekly Treat _____

You may be feeling... guilty for missing a session. Don't give yourself a hard time about it – that will simply make you feel bad and you'll be less likely to want to stick with the programme. Don't dwell on past mistakes – run away from them! There's nothing like simply getting out and running the next day to ease your conscience.

Week Eight

66 Success is the sum of small efforts, repeated day in and day out **99**
Robert Collier, self-help author

MONDAY Run 3 mins, walk 2 mins. Repeat 6 more times (Total: 35 mins)
Time of day you're planning to run:_____
Mood before: ☹ 😐 😏 😊 😃 Mood during: ☹ 😐 😏 😊 😃 Mood after: ☹ 😐 😏 😊 😃
Daily Reward _____

TUESDAY Rest

WEDNESDAY Try to increase your free session to 40 minutes – have fun!
Time of day you're planning to exercise:_____
Mood before: ☹ 😐 😏 😊 😃 Mood during: ☹ 😐 😏 😊 😃 Mood after: ☹ 😐 😏 😊 😃
Daily Reward _____

THURSDAY Rest

FRIDAY Run 3 mins, walk 2 mins. Repeat 6 more times (Total: 35 mins)
Time of day you're planning to run:_____
Mood before: ☹ 😐 😏 😊 😃 Mood during: ☹ 😐 😏 😊 😃 Mood after: ☹ 😐 😏 😊 😃
Daily Reward _____

SATURDAY Rest

SUNDAY Run 3 mins, walk 2 mins. Repeat 6 more times (Total: 35 mins)
Time of day you're planning to run:_____
Mood before: ☹ 😐 😏 😊 😃 Mood during: ☹ 😐 😏 😊 😃 Mood after: ☹ 😐 😏 😊 😃
Weekly Treat _____

You may be feeling... impatient, that the programme's holding you back rather than helping you move forward – but we promise it's not. What it's doing is making sure your body is ready to take running to another level, and that you aren't injured. We guarantee you'll get to run further once your body's ready, and that you'll be able to tackle races and even marathons (if you want a preview, check out Chapter Eight). Bear with us, because good things come to those who wait. You're well on your way to acquiring the exercise habit – which is even more important than simply getting fit.

❝ A man can succeed at almost anything for which he has unlimited enthusiasm ❞

Charles M Schwab, businessman

MONDAY Run 3 mins, walk 2 mins. Repeat 6 more times (Total: 35 mins)
Time of day you're planning to run:_____
Mood before: ☹ 😐 🙂 😊 😄 Mood during: ☹ 😐 🙂 😊 😄 Mood after: ☹ 😐 🙂 😊 😄
Daily Reward _____

TUESDAY Rest

WEDNESDAY Free session – 40 minutes of any activity you choose
Time of day you're planning to exercise:_____
Mood before: ☹ 😐 🙂 😊 😄 Mood during: ☹ 😐 🙂 😊 😄 Mood after: ☹ 😐 🙂 😊 😄
Daily Reward _____

THURSDAY Rest

FRIDAY Run 3 mins, walk 60 secs. Repeat 8 more times (Total: 36 mins)
Time of day you're planning to run:_____
Mood before: ☹ 😐 🙂 😊 😄 Mood during: ☹ 😐 🙂 😊 😄 Mood after: ☹ 😐 🙂 😊 😄
Daily Reward _____

SATURDAY Rest

SUNDAY Run 3 mins, walk 60 secs. Repeat 8 more times (Total: 36 mins)
Time of day you're planning to run:_____
Mood before: ☹ 😐 🙂 😊 😄 Mood during: ☹ 😐 🙂 😊 😄 Mood after: ☹ 😐 🙂 😊 😄
Weekly Treat _____

You may be feeling... slimmer. If weight loss was one of your goals, this should please you no end – and make you even more enthusiastic to finish the programme. Running is a fabulously efficient fat burner so by now you're likely to start seeing and feeling the difference. Book an appointment with your bank manager today – you're going to need an overdraft to finance your new wardrobe of sized-down clothes!

Week Ten

66 I celebrate myself 99
Walt Whitman, poet

MONDAY Run 3 mins, walk 60 secs. Repeat 8 more times (Total: 36 mins)
Time of day you're planning to run:_____
Mood before: ☹ ☹ ☺ ☺ ☺ Mood during: ☹ ☹ ☺ ☺ ☺ Mood after: ☹ ☹ ☺ ☺ ☺
Daily Reward _____

TUESDAY Rest

WEDNESDAY Free session – 40 minutes to do whatever exercise you like!
Time of day you're planning to exercise:_____
Mood before: ☹ ☹ ☺ ☺ ☺ Mood during: ☹ ☹ ☺ ☺ ☺ Mood after: ☹ ☹ ☺ ☺ ☺
Daily Reward _____

THURSDAY Rest

FRIDAY Run 3 mins, walk 60 secs. Repeat 8 more times (Total: 36 mins)
Time of day you're planning to run:_____
Mood before: ☹ ☹ ☺ ☺ ☺ Mood during: ☹ ☹ ☺ ☺ ☺ Mood after: ☹ ☹ ☺ ☺ ☺
Daily Reward _____

SATURDAY Rest

SUNDAY Run 3 mins, walk 60 secs. Repeat 9 more times (Total: 40 mins)
Time of day you're planning to run:_____
Mood before: ☹ ☹ ☺ ☺ ☺ Mood during: ☹ ☹ ☺ ☺ ☺ Mood after: ☹ ☹ ☺ ☺ ☺
Ultimate Indulgence!_____

You may be feeling… elated. And so you should! WELL DONE! You've reached your first goal and can now walk and run for up to 40 minutes – and should easily be able to complete a 5K (3-mile) race. Why not try a Race For Life – there are dozens all around the UK (visit www.raceforlife.org)? Isn't it amazing what a difference 60 seconds can make? Now treat yourself to that Ultimate Indulgence you've been promising yourself – you're a star and you deserve it.

'We tried it!'

We roped in two testers to put The 60-Second-Secret Plan through its paces – here's how they found it...

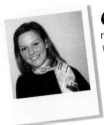

66 I've never been very good at PE or sticking to an exercise routine, so I was surprised to find myself really enjoying the plan. What I like the best is that it's easy to fit into your day. I also enjoyed the sessions while I was doing them, and by the second week was already having fantasies about running the London Marathon! It never felt hard to run for 60 seconds, though I did set off too fast in the first session and had to slow down my pace by the time I'd repeated the 60-second run a few times. Using the Mood-O-Meter proved to me just how much I was enjoying the sessions. Although on a few days I circled the Indifferent and Up And Down faces before my session, I always found myself circling the Good and Euphoric faces to sum up how great I felt while I was running along. For my rewards, I'd have a nice long soak in the bath before getting dressed up to go out for the night, or I'd watch *Sex And The City*.
Talia Wood, 21, journalism student, London 99

66 Before I started The 60-Second-Secret Plan, I hadn't run for three years because of a knee injury. When I first saw the programme, I thought, "Give me a break – I'm an international water-polo player and it's way too easy," but then I remembered that although I was fit, I'd barely run a step in three years. Secretly, I was very apprehensive about running again because I knew how hard it can be to start after a long lay-off. However, this programme made all the 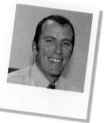 difference – I followed it to the letter (except for buying a sports bra and going dancing!) and I just couldn't believe how easily I got back into running. At times, I was tempted to run rather than walk but I kept reminding myself to take it slowly. I felt thrilled after each and every session as I went farther every time and, joy of joys, remained pain-free. I think men can be very competitive and may be reluctant to do something as unmanly as take a walk break, but I'm really glad I reined in that side of me. Having finished the programme, I'm now able to run 5km (3 miles) effortlessly and it's even made a difference to my water-polo as my legs are stronger.
Guy Mottram, 37, legal adviser, Johannesburg, South Africa 99

'How I got started'

Still feeling nervous about making your running debut? Remember, everyone was a beginner once. Take a look at how these runners got started, and then JUST DO IT!

66 I did my first run in Brighton when I was 20. I went downhill towards the sea, fast, in the wrong shoes, and ended up with sore shins. One good pair of shoes and mended shins later, I ran on the flat promenade, slowly, for what seemed like hours. Five minutes after I'd started, I arrived home. **My face was a terrifying colour, but I knew I was on to something**. And I was right. Fifteen years later, I'm still running. I've never run a race, nor do I aim to beat my times or run when I don't feel like it – because to me, running should be all about pleasure.' **Allie Packer, 35, journalist, London**

'When I turned 30, I thought the world had come to an end. **In a desperate attempt to ward off old age, I started running**. Clad in a white-and-brown minidress and tackies (tennis shoes), I became an odd but familiar sight in my neighbourhood at a time when running wasn't as popular among ordinary women as it is today. Thirty-three years later, I completed the New York City Marathon with my two daughters. My running gear has changed but that is about all. **Leone Jackson, 64, tour guide, Pretoria, South Africa**

'**Romance got me interested in running** at the ripe old age of 41. The woman in question was a very experienced runner and I tagged along to races with her just to have the chance to socialise with her afterwards. I'm now very much in love with running, and have done about 13,000km (more than 8,000 miles) worth of races. I'm also very much in love with Rina, whom I still run with and who's now my girlfriend!' **Pierre Jourdan, 53, technician, Pretoria, South Africa**

'I started running because **I was determined to lose weight**. Initially, I wobbled everywhere but now the extra 19kg (3st) I had put on has vanished and I'm trim and the happiest I've ever been. I know I'll never be Paula Radcliffe, but with running in my life, I'll always be a better version of me.'
Kat Arney, 27, scientist, London

'It was all the builders' fault! They came at 7.30am, in the middle of winter, too. I faced a stark choice – to sit in the kitchen huddled over a cup of tea or go for a walk. The walk won. After a few days, this seemed too slow and cold, so a faster shuffle was called for. **Before I knew it, I was running (slowly)**, round a 3km (2-mile) circuit. By the time the builders left, I was hooked. Four marathons later, I still ask myself why I do it. My family think I'm mad to lay myself open to blisters, black toenails and 42km (26.2 miles) of slog. But I guess the buzz I get from joining like-minded mad people in hurling ourselves down a road has to be experienced to be appreciated.'
Rosemary Beach, 63, tour guide, Oxford

'After an injury stopped me exercising for nearly a year, I took up running to try to regain some fitness, and also to get back in shape for my wedding day. I knew I wanted to start something I could maintain, and that wasn't just a quick fix, so I followed the walk/run plan in *Running Made Easy*.

For the first few weeks, I hated running so much that I had to repeat "fitter, slimmer, fitter, slimmer..." in my head to the rhythm of my running steps, to remind myself why on earth I was doing it! **I only had my 'breakthrough' moment in the fourth week of the plan,** when I absolutely loved every minute of my run, felt fantastic and truly enjoyed myself. Now I can't wait to go for my next run, and after I've been I feel happier and more positive and have more energy throughout the day.'
Charlotte Farrar, 28, Department of Health press officer, London

'Needing to do exercise of some sort, I joined a group of eight local long-distance runners and for 20 years **we ran together, doing runs that were filled with wonderful camaraderie, banter and reminiscences**. Even when some of us got too old to run, we continued to meet for dinner every two months. Now there are only two of us left but, along with our wives and two of the widows, we still meet as regularly and remember the others who have crossed the finish line before us. There's no doubt that my running years were a highlight of my life. The memories of all the hours together on the road with my friends, the happy nonsense that was talked and the experiences we shared, are still, and always will be, with me. **David Pistorius, 74, lawyer, Durban, South Africa**

'How I find the time to run'

Always got a million and one things competing for your time every day? Here, runners the world over tell you how they find time to run regularly despite their busy lives…

66 For me, the mornings are the best – **I get up early and run before work** when the air is fresh and the streets are quiet. It's quite a thrill getting into the office afterwards, knowing that you've already done your exercise for the day while most of your colleagues are still sipping their coffee, struggling to wake up.'
Carien du Plessis, 29, writer, Tasmania

'I love running **in the park at lunchtime** because it gives me a regular update of the seasons – in spring the daffodils and ducklings appear, in summer the tourists, then in autumn I watch the groundsmen blowing the leaves away. And winter brings the rain and snow.'
Alex Crowe, 29, IT support, London

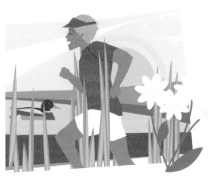

'My job with the police means I work different shifts, so I have to fit my running around them. I find that **going for a run outside in the fresh air and daylight really helps my head to clear and my body to adjust to waking and sleeping at different times** depending on whether I'm on an early shift or night duty. And I also find the variation in the times of day I run stops it becoming a monotonous routine.'
Sophie Easton, 33, crime scene examiner, the Metropolitan Police, Surrey

'My job means I find it very hard to make time to exercise. My day starts at 6.30am, and is packed full of back-to-back meetings, so **I don't get to go to the gym until about 9pm**. By then, I'm pretty tired but I tell myself that even if I manage only 10 minutes of running and a couple of stretches, I'll still have done well. What generally happens is that I start off with this thought and then keep adding 5 minutes extra until I've been running for 20 to 30 minutes. I know I'm playing little tricks on myself but they help me get started in the first place, which I think is the hardest part of exercise. After years of doing this, I also know that once I've done my "time", I really will feel like a whole new me!'
Justine Southall, 41, group publishing director, Surrey

'I've been **running to and from work** for about 30 years as it's the easiest way to make sure I fit running into my day. I've only forgotten to take in clothes to change into about twice – and on one of those occasions, a sympathetic cleaner lent me his tie for the day!' **John Collins, 66, manager, Swansea**

'The time that works for me is **straight after work**. I get changed at the salon, then go and run in Hyde Park. If I go home first and tell myself I'll run later in the evening, I always get distracted, start eating and make excuses not to go.' **Maria O'Keefe, 32, hair salon creative director, London**

'When I'm on a long car journey, rather than have a coffee break sitting in a service-station café, **I always plan my route so I can stop off and find a place like a park where I can run** – even if it's just for 15 minutes. The oxygen burst makes me feel much less tired and more relaxed for the second half of the journey.' **Michael Whalley, 62, teacher, Essex**

'I decided to make my long commute home more interesting by **running to the nearest Tube station**. It felt hard at first but after a few weeks I needed a new challenge and so ran to the next station on, before catching the Tube home from there. Then I began to add one Tube stop (about 1.6K/1 mile) to my run every week. Some day soon I'll be running all the way home (which is 21K/13 miles) – the equivalent of a half-marathon!' **Elizabeth Gowing, 29, education consultant, London**

'My job takes me all around the world, and **I throw my running gear into my suitcase even before my suit**. If I don't, I know I'll get that jittery feeling when 12 hours of sitting on the plane followed by eating way too much toxic restaurant food begin to make me crazy enough to want to run up the down escalator, slam-dance in the subway, anything to feel that endorphin high I get after a good run. When you're going insane in your hotel room and can't find a map, look in the phone book. A recent stay in the USA initially looked dismal, but the Yellow Pages revealed a park with many miles of riverside trails just beyond ugly industrial buildings. **Randy Brophy, 45, IT consultant, Sydney, Australia** 🙸

Do you want to learn how to make every run easier, more enjoyable and brilliant fun? We've road-tested advice from dozens of top experts and enthusiastic runners to bring you the 101 best-ever running tips of all time!

7

get the top tips

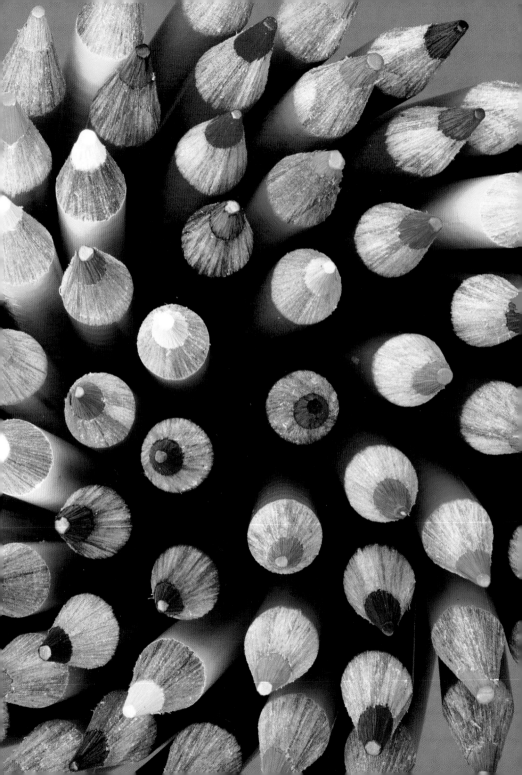

food & drink

1 **Don't panic!** You might think that if you take up running you have to junk whatever's in your cupboards and adopt a weird diet that revolves around endless pasta and sports drinks. Rest assured this isn't the case, especially when you're first starting out, says sports nutritionist Janet Thomson. 'As a beginner, you don't need to make radical changes to your diet, you just need to make sure you eat healthily and drink enough water,' she says. (However, if you really get bitten by the bug and start running like mad, you'll need to make some dietary changes, which we've covered in later tips.) So what counts as a healthy diet for total beginners? According to Sarah Schenker, a sports nutritionist at the British Nutrition Foundation, a healthy diet is a balanced one. 'One third of your intake should be made up of fruit and vegetables, one third made up of starchy carbohydrates (like pasta, potatoes, rice, breakfast cereals and bread) and then the remaining third should be divided up into three slices,' she explains. 'The largest slice (about 15%) should be milk and low-fat dairy foods, the second largest (about 12%) should be protein foods, such as meat, fish and vegetarian alternatives such as tofu, beans, pulses and eggs, and the final littlest slice (about 6%) should be left over for "naughty" foods that are higher in fat and sugar – chocolate, sweets and fizzy drinks all fall into this category.' Don't struggle to split every single meal precisely into these categories – the important thing is to achieve this kind of balance over a day, a week or a lifetime!

2 **Lose weight without trying** Get ready to make friends with food. Lots of people find that when they start running, they start making healthier eating choices, too. 'Taking up running gave me a natural push to think about changing my eating habits,' says Angela Charlemagne, 30, a graphic designer from London. 'I cut back loads on alcohol and fatty foods and instead started to eat more pasta, rice, fruit and veg. I lost about 3kg (7lb), and treated myself to a tasty pair of size 12 jeans to celebrate!'

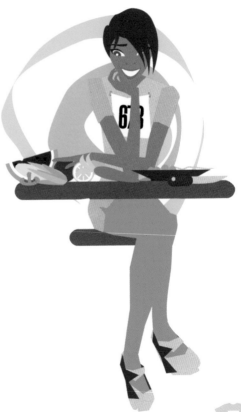

3 What to eat more of

While you don't have to change all your old habits, there are certain foods that are especially great for runners, and which you might like to start mixing into your diet. Here's a list of ten favourites from Liz Applegate, a sports nutritionist at the University of California, Davis, USA.

The top 10 runner's foods

✔ Salmon
✔ Lean red meat
✔ Soya-based veggie burgers
✔ Tofu
✔ Baked beans
✔ Breakfast cereal
✔ Sweet potatoes
✔ Wholewheat pasta
✔ Broccoli
✔ Brown rice

4 Drink plenty

Water is wonderful – make this your mantra and you can't go wrong as a new runner. Your body needs water for just about every function it has to perform, so making sure you begin your new running programme well hydrated will help get you feeling ready for anything! Here are some ways get you into the habit of drinking plenty each day...

⭐ 'I make sure I have a big glass of water first thing in the morning before I even have breakfast or start the school run,' says keen runner and mother of three Liza Robinson, 38, from Surrey. 'This helps jog my memory to keep drinking all day long – I can easily get so busy that I forget to drink completely.'

⭐ Buy a big bottle of water or fill a water jug and keep it on your desk so it reminds you to drink – take it to work meetings, too.

⭐ Drink little and often. Take sips in between phone calls or every time you come back to sit at your desk.

⭐ Fill smaller water bottles to keep with you during the day.

⭐ Be aware of how you feel when you've drunk plenty, so you really tap into the benefits. The chances are that you're clearer headed, more alert and more energetic.

⭐ Use the Pee Test to gauge how hydrated you are. If you've been drinking enough, your urine should be clear or pale and odourless. The darker and smellier it becomes, the less well hydrated you are.

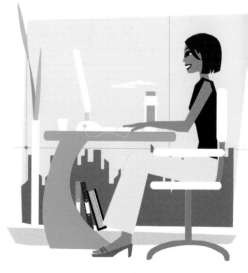

5 Eat carbs for energy

Carbohydrates are a runner's best friend because they're vital for giving you enough energy to exercise. As Shelly Vella, 37, marathon runner and fashion director of British *Cosmopolitan* magazine puts it, 'You can't run on empty – you only get back what you put in, which means it's so important to eat right. While I'm out running, I always take a banana with me in case I get hungry, and I always really look forward to my jacket potato when I get home.' Below we give some suggestions for which types of carb-based meals to eat and when, from nutritionist Clare Dodgshon of the Nutrition Matters Consultancy in London.

6 Experiment!

Although expert guidelines say you should eat 2 to 4 hours before exercise and top up with a smaller snack 1 hour to 30 minutes before, in reality, what works best can vary from person to person, says sports nutritionist Janet Thomson. 'I'd rather exercise an hour after eating than risk feeling hungry, because then I just can't function,' she says. However, runner and sports PR consultant Jane Cowmeadow, 39, is just the opposite. 'I'm definitely someone who can't eat much before a run,' she says. 'I train every Saturday morning at 11am, and only have a couple of digestive biscuits and a mug of tea an hour or two beforehand, then save myself for a big brunch afterwards.'

||||➡ KNOW YOUR CARBS

For your pre-run meal Try a chicken, prawn, tuna or cheese sandwich on granary bread, a jacket potato or granary toast with baked beans or tuna, a portion of sushi, or pasta with vegetables and tomato sauce, followed by yogurt or a handful of dried fruit such as apricots.

For your pre-run snack If your last meal was more than 2 hours ago, have a snack half an hour before your run to give you a fast energy rush. Try a slice of white toast with jam, a mini fruit scone, a couple of rice cakes, or a glass of diluted fruit juice.

During your run If you'll be running for longer than 60 to 90 minutes, drink an isotonic sports drink (see tip 11), otherwise stick to water.

After your run If you're going to run quite hard again the next day, snack within 30 minutes of finishing. Try honey sandwiches, white or wholemeal toast, or a bowl of cereal. Then eat a meal within 2 hours, making it a good balance of carbs and protein. Try potatoes or brown rice with meat, fish, lentils, pulses or tofu and vegetables.

7 Bring a bottle

Bring a bottle After slipping into a good sports bra and trainers, your next don't-go-running-without-it essential is a little bottle of water clutched in your hand. Plain water is all you need for any run that's less than an hour long – aim to sip about 125ml to 250ml (a quarter to a half-pint, or about 7 to 14 swallows!) every 10 to 20 minutes during exercise, says top sports nutritionist Anita Bean. But don't fall into the trap of drinking excessive amounts of water, as this can bring on a potentially very dangerous condition called hyponatremia or water intoxication, when your blood is diluted so much that sodium levels fall, making you feel dizzy and causing breathing problems. 'Some longer-distance, slower runners in particular can tend to take in huge amounts of water,' says Dr Dan Tunstall Pedoe, medical director of the Flora London Marathon, 'and then end up collapsing after a race. You need to realise that drinking too much can be as problematic as drinking too little.'

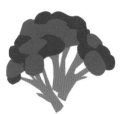

8 Eat more antioxidants

Eat more antioxidants One of the very, very few drawbacks of exercise is that it increases your production of free radicals, which are unstable molecules that rampage around your body causing harm to healthy cells. Luckily, there's an easy way to fight back – by eating more antioxidant-rich foods, which are not only delicious but disarm the nasty free radicals, rendering them harmless. Below is a top-ten list of favourites complied by US-based sports nutritionist Liz Applegate.

Top 10 antioxidant foods and drinks

- ✔ Strawberries
- ✔ Oranges
- ✔ Chocolate (dark or milk)
- ✔ Green or black tea
- ✔ Red wine (in moderation)
- ✔ Broccoli
- ✔ Tomatoes
- ✔ Spinach
- ✔ Carrots
- ✔ Dried apricots

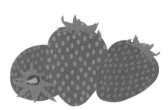

9 Befriend your bowels

If you're someone who suffers from constipation, here's the good news – running is an amazing, drug-free solution that should help get things moving down there again! But be warned, some people find running shakes things up a bit too much, making them need to go to the loo suddenly and urgently while they're out running (something that's affectionately known as getting 'runner's trots'). The good news is that this doesn't have to put you off. Here are some coping strategies...

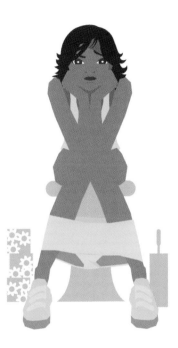

||||▶ Start by running somewhere with public toilets so you can gauge the effect that running has on you. After a couple of weeks, you'll know what to expect – and when! 'I always need the loo 20 minutes into a run, and then once I've been, I'm absolutely fine for the rest of the time,' says one runner. 'I just need to make sure my first loop of the park ends up outside the Ladies!'

||||▶ Experiment with what you eat beforehand – lots of runners find high-fibre cereal causes problems before an earl morning run, and are better off just having toast, or running on an empty stomach. 'If I had cereal with milk before a run, I'd always end up having to call my boyfriend to come and get me in the car and whizz me home to the loo,' says one novice runner who found dairy products a particular trigger.

||||▶ Try a cup of tea or coffee to help get your bowels moving before you set off on your run.

10 Write a success recipe

Keep a food diary for a few weeks, especially if you're new to running. Write down which meals and snacks you had and how close to your run, plus how they made you feel. This should help you gauge what does and doesn't agree with you. For example, if you tried eating dried apricots on several occasions before your run and ended up with stomach ache every time, you'll know to avoid them in future. Going back over your diary will enable you to write a recipe for running success.

11 Go-farther drinks

If you want to start running for longer than about 60 to 90 minutes, it's time to enter the wonderful world of sports drinks. These not only rehydrate you, they also top up your energy levels. 'Look out for a drink that's called isotonic, which means it has the same concentration of carbohydrates and mineral salts you'd find in your body's own fluids, and so is absorbed as fast as or faster than plain water,' says sports nutritionist Anita Bean. 'Most ready-made isotonic drinks contain between 4g and 8g of carbohydrates per 100ml (3½ oz) of fluid, and you could drink up to one litre (or a little less than two pints) of them an hour,' she says, 'though this might be too much for some people. Drinks like Lucozade Sport or Gatorade will tend to be a bit more concentrated and so a bit more calorific, so you can choose to make your own if you want

something more diluted. Experiment, as different drinks suit different people. Just don't try something brand new on an important run or race day!'

To make your own: Fill your water bottle half-full with pure orange or apple juice, then top it up with water. This will give you a slightly more dilute, and less calorific, isotonic drink with a concentration of about 5g to 6g of carbs per 100ml (3½ oz). If this is still too strong, experiment by watering it down even more.

12 Go-faster foods

Want to discover a secret ingredient that can help you to run faster? Then try omega-3 fatty acids. They're a type of essential fatty acid most of us really don't get enough of, but which improve the delivery of oxygen to our body's cells, increasing our energy levels and stamina. Get the right amount by eating one portion of oily fish such as mackerel, herrings, sardines, salmon or fresh tuna every week (pregnant women should limit consumption of tuna owing to the mercury it contains). One omega-3-enriched egg (Columbus eggs) or a medium-sized sweet potato also meet your daily needs. Or try having two tablespoons of omega-3-rich linseeds with your normal bowl of cereal every morning. Soak them in a little water overnight to make it easier for your body to absorb their goodness, and then add the seeds with the water to your cereal. But for some people, they can have the kind of go-faster effect that gets you sprinting for the toilet, so don't eat them too close to a run!

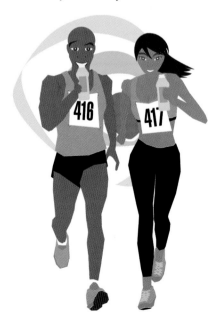

13 **Create a snack stash** It's almost impossible to motivate yourself to go out running if you're hungry before you even start. Squirrel away some healthy treats so you've always got a little something to eat before a run – and keep snacks to hand when you finish so you don't end up starving and miles from your next meal. See right for some great and tasty options, as recommended by accredited sports dietician Jacqueline Boorman...

14 **Swig from the start** If you're running a longer race like a half- or full marathon, start drinking your sports drink in the early to mid part of the race – not just as the finish line comes into sight! This will give it the 20 or so minutes it needs to raise your blood-sugar levels and give you a much-needed energy burst.

15 **Eat to beat injuries** Don't just eat for energy – eat to beat aches and pains, as well. The foods below can help to keep you supple and injury free:

||||▶ Antioxidant-rich foods
You need good supplies of foods rich in the antioxidant vitamins C and E, because studies have found they help banish post-workout soreness faster. They work their magic by battling against the nasty free radicals that are produced after exercise, and which cause muscle soreness. Getting your five portions of fruit and vegetables a day will keep your antioxidant levels nice and high, as will eating certain

The top 10 runner's snacks

✔ Banana
✔ Low-fat yogurt and piece of fruit
✔ Toasted bagel with Marmite, jam or peanut butter
✔ Fruit smoothie made with milk or yogurt
✔ 2 to 3 fresh Medjool dates
✔ Bowl of plain popcorn
✔ Slice of fruit loaf or malt loaf
✔ Handful of pretzels
✔ Handful of dried fruit – raisins, apricots, figs, tropical-fruit mix
✔ 2 to 3 Jaffa cakes

other foods (see tip 8), but you can also top yours up with a good antioxidant supplement.

||||▶ Omega-3-rich foods
These earn another brownie point for their anti-inflammatory properties, and help both to prevent injuries and speed healing, says Anita Bean (see tip 12 for good sources).

16 **Get steamy** Steam rather than boil your veggies – it'll help to conserve more of the vitamins, minerals and precious antioxidants your body needs when you're a runner.

17 Eat chocolate

Take a tip from marathon world-record holder Paula Radcliffe and try eating a few squares of milk chocolate (she favours Dairy Milk) before a race to give you a delicious and sustained energy boost. Or, if you're someone who can eat on the run, save it for a certain point in the race so you have something lovely to look forward to!

18 Be a good mixer

Eating protein (meat, eggs, tofu) at the same time as carbohydrates (bread, pasta, potatoes) helps you stay fuller for longer and does your muscles big favours, too, says Craig Copland, a sports-nutrition adviser for nutrition company EAS. 'The carbs make your body release the hormone insulin, which acts like a key, opening the cells to allow them to absorb the amino acids contained in the protein, which are essential for muscle repair.' Try a ham, cheese or chicken sandwich; peanut butter on toast; pasta or rice with chicken, tofu or soya; or a baked potato topped with cottage cheese.

19 How to diet and run

Running is a brilliant fat burner, which can help you shed the pounds and shape up fast. If you're taking up a basic running programme (see Chapter Six) and want to cut back on calories without sapping your energy levels, 400 calories is a good amount to shave from your daily intake, says dietitian and weight-loss expert Lyndel Costain. This, along with the increase in your activity levels, should get you

losing weight (and especially body fat) at the steady and sustainable rate of about 450g (1lb) a week. 'If you have some weight to lose, you're likely to have been eating at least 2,000 calories a day before you started running,' says Costain. 'This means you'll now have about 1,600 to 1,700 calories to allocate between your meals, your drinks and pre-run snacks. Timing really is key to making sure you don't get too hungry, or feel too tired to run. Aim to eat little and often so you can fit in three meals and two to three snacks a day – this helps keep your blood-sugar levels stable, energy levels up and hunger at bay.'

See Your Weight-Loss Eating Plan, right, for ideas on how to allocate your calories throughout the day...

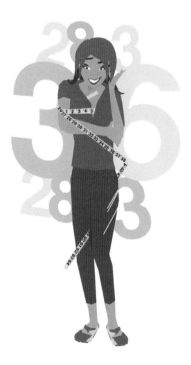

YOUR WEIGHT-LOSS EATING PLAN

If you're trying to lose weight but still want the energy to run, here's how you could split your calories…

350-calorie breakfast
A medium-sized bowl of cereal with skimmed milk, plus one slice of wholegrain toast and low-fat spread. You also need to drink plenty of water to stay well hydrated.

100-calorie milk allowance
In addition to the skimmed milk you had on your cereal, this plan also includes 200ml (7fl oz) of semi-skimmed milk that you can use in up to four or five cups of tea or coffee (but make sure you don't have them with lots of sugar). If you drink your tea or coffee black, swap the milk for a 200g (7oz) pot of low-fat yogurt.

100-calorie mid-morning snack
A large banana or three rice cakes or two oat cakes.

350-calorie lunch
Bowl of lentil and vegetable soup, plus a slice of wholegrain toast, plus a pot of low-fat yogurt (in addition to the optional one above), plus a piece of fruit.

150-calorie pre-run snack eaten 30 to 60 minutes before your run
A fruit bun or large handful of dried fruit or cereal bar or small pot of rice pudding. Drink water if you're running for less than an hour; if you're going for longer, use an isotonic sports drink or make up diluted pure orange juice with an equal amount of water. Note the calorie content, though – 500ml (about a pint) of either drink will provide about 100 calories that you may want to trim from elsewhere, or leave as is (the extra running will help compensate for it).

150-calorie post-run snack
A shop-bought smoothie or small packet of nuts and raisins or cereal with semi-skimmed milk or half a bagel topped with low-fat cream cheese.

400-calorie dinner
Stir-fried rice or noodles with chicken, fish or tofu, plus plenty of vegetables.

TOTAL: 1,600 calories, or 1,700 if you opted for the isotonic drink or diluted orange juice.

20 How to carbo-load

You've probably heard marathon runners justify their huge pasta and cake intake just before a big race by explaining they're 'carbo-loading', but what's the point of all this feasting, and do you really need to do it? Basically, carbo-loading is all about feeding your body with lots of carbohydrate, so it can turn it into an energy source called glycogen, which it stores in your muscles and liver and uses to keep you going during the race. The goal is to super-charge your glycogen stores before you set off on a race, thus enabling you to keep going for longer before they run out. So how do you do it? In the week leading up to the race, simply ease back on the amount of running you're doing, and eat slightly more carbohydrates, but don't use it as an excuse to binge! 'It's best to eat a few more carbs without going mad,' says sports nutrition expert Professor Ron Maughan at Loughborough University. 'If you overdo it, you'll gain weight, which isn't helpful, and having a lot more glycogen doesn't bring huge benefits. Your performance is much more dictated by your training.'

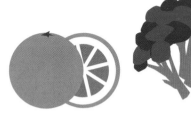

21 Pump up your iron intake

'Iron deficiency is the most common deficiency I see in runners, as you lose iron through sweating,' says accredited sports dietician Jacqueline Boorman. 'The impact of your feet hitting the ground as you run also destroys red blood cells. This means it's very important to eat an iron-rich diet to keep your iron stores topped up. I'm very pro red meat as animal sources of iron are easier for your body to absorb. Try to have lean beef, liver (but not if you're pregnant), lamb or exotic options such as venison or ostrich at least twice a week. If you're vegetarian, you have to work harder to get your iron so eat iron-rich foods every day. Good choices are iron-enriched breakfast cereals, beans, nuts, seeds and lentils, eggs and green vegetables, especially spinach and broccoli. Because the iron from vegetarian sources is harder for your body to absorb, eat them with a glass of orange juice, as the vitamin C aids iron absorption. And try to avoid drinking tea with your vegetarian meal because it hinders absorption.' If you suspect you're anaemic – signs include getting more breathless than normal during your runs and feeling tired all the time despite sleeping well – ask your doctor to do a blood test to check.

22 There's no magic formula!

Top athletes experiment with their diets for years, tweaking what, when and how much they eat to keep on getting better results – and no identical magic formula works for any two of them. They're all highly individual. Take a leaf from their book and don't expect to get your eating right overnight – you can keep learning for the whole of your running life.

23 Porridge power

If you tend to feel queasy or even throw up after you've run hard, try eating something small such as a cereal bar the moment you finish your run. It seems to help settle the stomach. And, before your run, try porridge. One theory is that you feel sick because of dehydration, and if you eat a food such as porridge that contains plenty of fluid, it helps by giving you a constant supply.

24 It's OK to tipple...

There's no reason why running should turn you teetotal – it's fine to carry on drinking in moderation as long as you get your timing right. 'Don't drink alcohol at lunchtime if you're going for an evening run,' says Sarah Schenker, a sports nutritionist at the British Nutrition Foundation, 'and don't drink straight after a race when your body hasn't had a chance to rehydrate. But otherwise, stick to safe drinking guidelines and you'll be fine.' Women are advised to have no more than two to three units a day, and men no more than three to four units a day. At least one alcohol-free day each week is also a good idea for both sexes. (One unit equals a 125ml glass of wine, a standard pub measure of spirits, or half a pint of average-strength beer.) 'I cut down on the amount of alcohol I drank while I was training for the London Marathon because I didn't like trying to run with a hangover,' says Louise Longman, 30, a journalist from London, 'but I couldn't have given it up altogether. I had a glass of red wine with my pasta the night before the race, and it really helped me relax and get a good night's sleep before the big day.'

25 ... but don't run with a hangover

'This is because the alcohol can raise your blood pressure and will dehydrate you, both of which could contribute to heart problems if you try to "run off" a hangover,' warns cardio expert Dr Dorian Dugmore of Wellness International at Adidas.

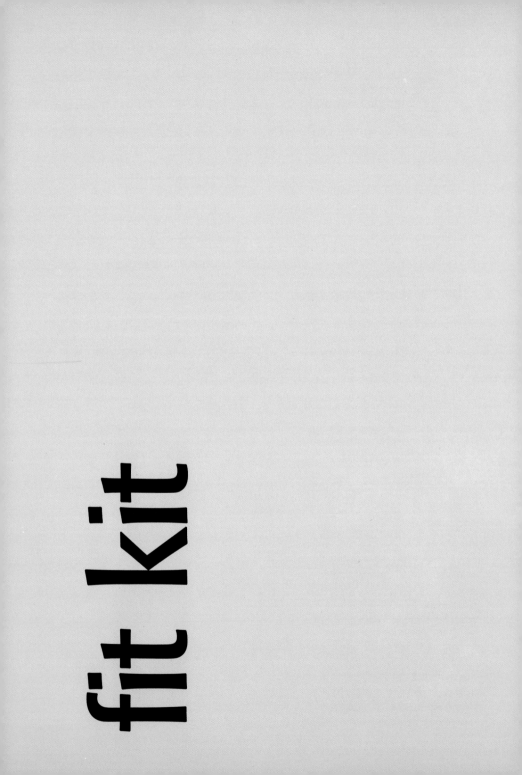

fit kit

26 Let's go shopping

So you're in a sports shop and your credit card's burning a hole in your pocket – what do you need to know?

★ 'There are two important things to look out for when choosing running gear – comfort and moisture management,' says Brian Connell, running category manager for Nike. 'Clothing should be comfortable and well tailored so that loose pieces of material don't flap or catch. For moisture management, choose a fabric such as Nike's Dri-FIT, which "wicks" [draws] sweat away from your body so it can evaporate, thus keeping you dry.' Other wicking fabrics include Adidas's CoolMax and Reebok's Playdry.

★ If your thighs rub together and wear holes in your running shorts when you run, slip into something more comfortable – Lycra! One runner we know was getting through a pair of shorts every three months until she switched to Lycra – she has now had the same ones for years. (An oversized T-shirt will cover any lumpy bits the Lycra may reveal.)

★ If you sweat heavily, seek out sportswear containing a fab new antibacterial fibre called X-STATIC. This contains pure silver, which kills 99.9% of odour-causing bacteria. X-STATIC also draws sweat away from your skin and is thermo-regulating, so it'll keep you warm in winter and cool in summer.

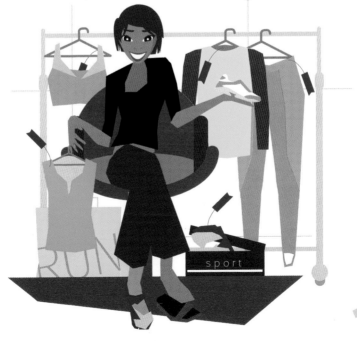

27 Feet first

Choosing the correct trainers is the single most important decision you'll make in your running career. Get it right and you'll be protected against injury and enjoy hundreds of miles of pain-free, smooth running. Get it wrong and you'll be exposing yourself to all sorts of problems. Here's some advice on making the right choice:

★ Always go to a specialist running shop, not a high-street fashion store. You need expert advice, not the trainers being worn by the latest boy band.

★ The best time of day to go shoe shopping is in the afternoon, after you've been walking about, because your feet will be at their biggest then.

★ Take along any trainers you've been running in (they may help the salesperson assess your running style), as well as the socks you'll be wearing to run.

★ Shoe shopping shouldn't be done in a rush. Try on lots of different trainers so you can get a good feel for what's most comfortable. Buy only trainers that feel totally comfortable from the word go, or you'll have miles of misery trying to wear them in.

★ Don't skimp on what you spend – expect to pay at least £60. Running is a very inexpensive sport (there are no gym fees to pay and you need minimal equipment), so you can afford to splash out a bit on your trainers.

28 Insole searching

Orthotics (also known as orthoses) are thin, sole-like inserts that you slip into your trainers to iron out any kinks in the way your feet function in order to help you run more efficiently. For example, an orthotic can help stabilise your foot and ankle, or if one leg is longer than the other, it can be used to 'lengthen' your shorter leg.

Who needs orthotics? 'They're only vital for about 10% of people,' says Simon Costain, a podiatrist at the Gait and Posture Centre in Harley Street, London, 'but about 75% of people could also benefit from using them. If you develop a running injury that won't go away even though you've been to see a physio, you may find it helpful to see a podiatrist who will watch you move to determine whether your injury stems from a biomechanical imbalance and can be put right with some expert advice and the use of orthotics.' To find a podiatrist near you, visit www.feetforlife.org.

29 Test yourself

Although staff at a specialist running shop will be highly trained and ready to help you select your perfect running shoe, it's also a good idea (and quite fun) to get to know your feet beforehand, so you go in with a rough idea of the kind of shoes you should be buying. Sean Fishpool, British *Runner's World*'s shoe expert, suggests doing The Wet-Footprint Test (see opposite) …

⥤ THE WET-FOOTPRINT TEST

Step out of the bath or shower on to a piece of cardboard or a dark towel, then compare the imprint you leave with those below...

You have a...	So you're likely to be...	So choose...
Normal/ neutral foot	**a normal pronator**, in other words, your foot lands on the outer side of your heel and then rolls slightly inwards before you push off on the ball of your foot and your toes. This means your foot is a good shock-absorber	trainers in the **stability** category
Flat foot	**an overpronator**, in other words, your foot lands on the outer side of your heel but then rolls inwards (or pronates) too much before you push off on the ball of your foot and your toes, which can lead to running injuries	trainers in the **motion-control** category
High-arched foot	**a supinator**, in other words, your foot lands on the outer side of your heel but doesn't roll inwards enough before you push off on the ball of your foot and your toes. This means your foot isn't a very good shock-absorber	trainers in the **cushioned** category

30 Resist those rays

As a runner, you'll be spending a lot more time outdoors than most people, so wearing a sunscreen, during both summer and winter, is a must. Use it each and every time you go out in daylight – even if it's overcast, sunshine can still penetrate cloud. And remember to reapply it frequently, especially on the back of your neck and your ears. Choose one that protects against both UVA and UVB rays with an SPF of at least 15 – and preferably much higher than that if you live in a very hot climate, says Dr Lewis Maharam, medical director of the New York City Marathon. 'It's also very important to choose one that's non-greasy and specifically formulated to allow you to sweat, as sunscreens that stop you perspiring can increase your risk of heatstroke,' he adds.

He recommends looking for products such as Banana Boat Sport Sunblock Lotion and Coppertone Oil Free Sunblock Lotion.

A hat or cap will also shield you from the sun (one that covers the back of your neck is a good idea) and sunglasses will help protect your eyes (and make you look seriously sporty!). Wear loose, lightweight clothing that covers your upper arms. On very hot days, avoid running between 10am and 4pm when the sun's at its hottest and remember that you'll need to drink extra fluids to compensate for all the extra sweating you're going to be doing. You should also pour water over yourself or use a wet sponge to cool yourself down while you're out.

'If you experience dizziness, weakness, headache, disorientation and a lack of coordination and your skin feels cold and clammy, you may be suffering from heat exhaustion,' says Professor Clyde Williams, professor of sports science at Loughborough University. 'In this case, you should stop running at once, seek out some shade, drink a sports drink, some rehydration mixture or water with a little salt in it, and use water to cool your body down rapidly.'

31 Layer on up

'Remember the 20-degree rule!' (which works for Fahrenheit but not Celsius) says Rachael Beach, 31, a graphic artist from Bicester. 'You'll always be a lot hotter than you think, so if it's 50°F outside, once you start running you'll feel as if it's 70°F. So dress in layers that you can strip off. For spectators, however, it'll always feel 20°F colder, so wrap up warm!'

32 Dress down

When you've got new kit, don't throw away your old clothes just yet – they may come in handy at races. Many events involve standing around in the early morning chill, so having an old sweatshirt to wear (and that you can discard once you've warmed up after the first couple of miles) can be a real godsend. Many runners also swear by bin bags, which are highly portable and, with the simple addition of a few holes for your arms and head, will keep you toasty and dry. Who cares if it's not your most glam moment?

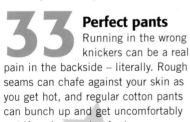

33 Perfect pants

Running in the wrong knickers can be a real pain in the backside – literally. Rough seams can chafe against your skin as you get hot, and regular cotton pants can bunch up and get uncomfortably wet if you're running for longer distances. It's worth buying some of the special sporty pants coming onto the market. They're not cheap, but they're comfortable, seam-free and breathable. We think they're worth every penny.

34 Get greasy!

Guys, unless you want to finish a race looking as if someone's painted two red bull's-eyes on the front of your T-shirt, apply copious amounts of Vaseline to your nipples (plasters also do the trick). 'I was advised by a friend who'd already run lots of races to rub Vaseline on my nipples,' says Dermot Fitzpatrick, 47, a runner and signwriter from Glasgow. 'Because I thought he was joking, I didn't bother, and eventually the constant chafing against my T-shirt made my nipples bleed. After that, I always slathered on plenty and they were fine.' Also slap on Vaseline anywhere you're likely to get chafed, such as in your groin and under your arms, under your water-bottle belt strap and around your bra straps.

35 Don't brace yourself

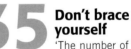

'The number of people who wear knee bandages and braces is incredible,' says Dr Dan Tunstall Pedoe, medical director of the Flora London Marathon. 'They may alter the pull of muscles slightly, but at best they're simply a psychological crutch.' Spend your money instead on finding out what's causing the pain by going to see your GP, a physiotherapist, an osteopath or a podiatrist (orthotics may help, see tip 28).

36 If the shoe fits...

Try before you buy should be your motto when shopping for trainers, says Shankara Smith, manager of legendary London running shop

Run And Become. It's perfectly acceptable to ask if you can run up and down outside the shop – many stores will send an expert with you to watch and assess if you're in the right shoes. While running, check whether the shoes feel too loose or tight. Many runners need to wear trainers one or more sizes larger than normal – when standing up, allow a half to a full thumb's width of space between your longest toe and the tip of the shoe, otherwise your toes will slam against the end of the trainers, resulting in black toenails. You may be a different size in different brands of trainers, so do the thumb test with each pair. To check whether your shoes fit widthwise, look at how far apart the lace eyelets are when you're wearing them – if they're two finger-widths apart, that's ideal.

37 Get plastered!

Friction between your skin and your running shoes or socks causes blisters. 'Anything that intensifies rubbing can cause them, such as wet socks, ill-fitting trainers or running longer distances, which will make your feet swell,' says Lorraine Jones, a state-registered podiatrist/chiropodist. Wearing well-fitting trainers and double-layered or moisture-wicking socks (which draw sweat away from your skin) can help prevent blisters, as can turning seamed socks inside out and coating your feet with Vaseline, says Jones. You can also try using blister plasters (such as those made by Compeed) on blister-prone areas.

38 Buy a bestseller

When choosing trainers, it pays to go for a big-name brand. Susie is a big fan of Asics trainers and has run all her marathons in them, but also rates trainers by Nike, while Lisa loves Adidas and New Balance trainers, which she says make her feel 'bouncy like Tigger'!

To give you an idea of how the top brands compare, we asked James Morris, manager of top running store Sweatshop in Teddington, to come up with a list of the bestselling brands through his shop. His customers certainly know their stuff, and include Olympic medallist Sonia O'Sullivan, and elite British athlete Mo Farah. We've given each brand's website so you can go online and get an idea of the shoes they offer before you make your trip to a shop to get fitted. However, unless you've

Bestselling brands

1. ASICS
www.asics.co.uk
2. NIKE
www.nike.com
3. BROOKS
www.brooksrunning.com
4. MIZUNO
www.mizunoeurope.com
5. SAUCONY
www.saucony.com
6. NEW BALANCE
www.newbalance.co.uk
7. ADIDAS
www.adidas.com
8. PUMA
www.pumarunning.com

bought a particular trainer before and know it suits you, don't order from the internet without trying – it's an expensive way to make mistakes!

39 Go-faster fit kit
Excitingly enough, you can now find kit specifically designed to enable you to run faster and smarter. Here's a few of our favourite options:

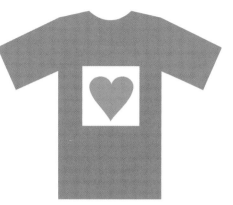

- Inner Muscle Technology clothing from Asics is a range of kit designed to work hard-to-target 'inner muscles' you never even knew you had! The theory is that by wearing clothes that work these muscles for you, your posture, running speed and efficiency will improve. And Asics has evidence to back their claims — 70% of people who wore the Inner Muscle Training Tight (which looks like a pair of regular cycling shorts) walked with a longer stride, and 80% had an increase in muscle strength, which meant they could lift their knees more strongly.
- We're also impressed by compression clothing from a brand called 2XU. Basically, it's tight-fitting gear, designed to do a range of things including reduce how much your muscles vibrate during exercise. This in turn improves muscle endurance and strength. Studies claim this could help a 3:30 marathon runner knock 5 minutes off their time – and it certainly seems to work for Paula Radcliffe, who wears compression socks. But the clothing isn't just for the elite runner; because it

wraps muscles tightly, and helps flush out the waste products that build up during exercise more quickly, it's also great for reducing the aches and pains and injuries beginners can tend to suffer.

40 Prepare for pit stops! Always carry
some tissues or loo roll with you, and before you go on a long run, work out where all the potential loo stops are along the route. Loos and loo roll are important as the bouncing motion of running, dehydration, pre-race nerves and even lactose (milk) intolerance can all cause an urgent need to dash to the loo to void your bowels. If you're worried about needing to go when there's no loo in sight, tuck a small cloth into your knickers for peace of mind.

A sanitary pad or cloth will also help with another problem that many women face when running, especially after pregnancy – urinary incontinence. However, doing pelvic floor exercises as often as possible can help put a stop to this. While standing, sitting or lying down, simply contract your pelvic floor muscles (as if you were trying to stop peeing in mid-flow), hold for a few seconds, then release for a few seconds. Repeat for up to 5 minutes a few times a day.

41 Bra-vo! A good sports bra is the only way to ensure running doesn't become a pain in the bust (many larger-chested runners swear by wearing two!). Don't delay, get one (or two) today. Lack of support can result in stretched breast ligaments and irreversible sagging. A study at Heriot-Watt University in Edinburgh, Scotland, found that wearing a sports bra reduced breast movement by 56%.

Here's what to look out for when you go bra buying:

* Running counts as a high-impact exercise, so select sports bras labelled high impact, or check the back of the box to see if they're suitable for running.
* Once you've got the bra on, your breasts should feel securely flattened against your chest – but the bra shouldn't be so tight that it stops you breathing! Have an experimental jump up and down on the spot to see if you're going to jiggle. Check the feel of the straps, too – are they wide enough? Do they feel as if they'll slip?

42 Bless your cotton socks Many runners, ourselves included, are happy to run in cotton socks as long as they're not too short (so they don't slip down into your

shoes) and fit snugly (so they don't wrinkle and cause blisters). But make sure you get the seams straight – if they're twisted, they'll rub and cause blisters. However, if your feet sweat heavily or you're going for a long run, cotton may not be for you as it absorbs moisture and swells, rubbing against your skin to cause blisters. Instead, you may want to opt for socks made from acrylic, polyester, Tactel or CoolMax/Dri-FIT (fabrics that draw moisture away from your skin). If you're blister-prone, try 'blister-free' double-layered socks.

43 Have a heart-rate monitor These measure your heart rate and can help you assess whether you're training too hard or whether you're having the equivalent of a lie-in when you're out running! Many runners swear by brands such as Polar, but, if you're the non-techie type who's never quite figured out how to programme your DVD player, you may find them more trouble than they're worth.

44 Smart shoes At the very high end of the kit market, top brands compete to surpass themselves by offering ever more sophisticated running trainers. One ultra-smart model is the adidas_1 DLX Runner, dubbed 'the shoe with a brain'. It contains a motor, sensor and microprocessor that receives information on your running pace, style and the surface you're running on, so it can continually adapt the level of cushioning you need.

45 Drugs that don't work (and ones that do)

Don't be tempted to take a painkiller before a race to head off any aches and pains that may surface during it. 'This isn't a very good idea,' says pharmacist Maeve O'Connell, 'as pain is your body's way of telling you something's wrong and this will simply drown out the messages it's trying to send you. Get to the bottom of the pain instead by going to see a health professional.'

However, if you're in a lot of pain during the course of a race, 'try taking paracetamol (brand names Panadol, Solpadeine and Syndol),' says Dr Lewis Maharam, medical director of the New York City Marathon. 'Avoid non-steroidal anti-inflammatories such as ibuprofen (brand names Advil and Nurofen) and aspirin (brand names Disprin, Aspirin and Aspro) when you're running as they can decrease blood flow to your kidneys and therefore prevent proper salt metabolism. This is an additional risk factor for a condition known as hyponatremia (an abnormally low concentration of sodium in your blood, which in very extreme cases can be fatal, see tip 7). Taking them when not running, however, is fine.'

46 Safely does it

Remember, you're hoping that running will prolong your life, not radically curtail it, so always keep safety at the front of your mind when you're out.

- Don't cross roads when the traffic lights are red – jog on the spot until they turn green again.
- Never run outdoors with an iPod, as it'll prevent you hearing approaching traffic.
- Avoid running on your own in deserted areas (run with a big dog or a friend instead) and stick to well-lit, populated areas if running at night. Consider running with a rape alarm.

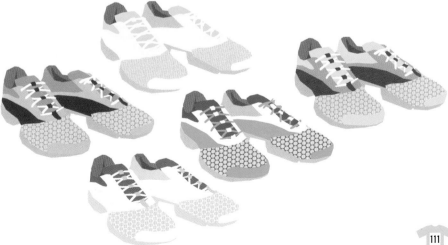

⭐ Always carry some form of identification with an emergency contact number, a phone card, small change and enough money for a bus or taxi ride home just in case you get injured. If you have any type of serious medical condition, wear a MedicAlert bracelet or carry written information about it with you.

⭐ Let someone know the route you'll be taking and what time you expect to get back (write a note and put it up on your fridge if you live alone or no one's at home when you set out). Vary your route and the time when you run to avoid someone trailing you.

⭐ 'If people shout comments at you when you're out running,' says Mailynne Woolley, 43, an art director from Maidenhead, 'maintain a contemptuous silence and avoid eye contact. Whatever you do, don't let it bug you or ruin your run. Those people are more than likely just feeling guilty that they're not out running themselves.'

47 Move to the beat

When iPod fever swept the globe, it changed how we listen to music for ever, and now it's also changing the way we run. Apple and Nike have teamed up to produce 'Nike+'; a package designed to give you music, information and motivation in one go. At the heart of Nike+ is a special chip that fits into your trainer and communicates with your iPod nano, so as well as getting music through your headphones, you get information on how far and fast you've run and how many calories you've burned. It also links into a website (www.nikeplus.com) where you can log your runs, and chat with other runners.

48 Hit the bottle

Running shops stock all manner of water bottles (plus rucksacks and belts to carry them in), so take your pick. Make sure you can run entirely comfortably holding one and that you wash it frequently in hot, soapy water. If you don't like carrying water with you, make sure you've noted where all the likely watering points are on your intended route (water fountains, taps, public toilets, pubs).

49 Be bright

Making yourself visible to passing traffic is the secret to a happy road-running career. If you're running in the dark, wear light-reflective clothes and shoes like Stewart Granby, 45, an accounting manager from Shorashim in Israel. 'Running round the city streets at night is a dangerous pastime,' he says. 'Many Israeli drivers are very impatient and no one, not even poor, defenceless runners, will stop them from getting to their final destination in the shortest possible time. At night I wear a light-coloured vest and a reflective strip across my chest and back. I'm very alert when I run and make sure I'm always aware of what the traffic's doing.'

50 Baby, it's cold outside

There are just three things you have to remember when running in the cold: layers, layers, layers. It's far easier to remove a layer and tie it round your waist than it is to run home to fetch one! Here are some tips on how to layer up.

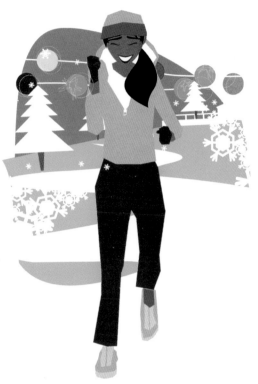

IIII▶ Upper body You may need up to three layers:

Inner layer This needs to be a breathable fabric, such as Nike's Dri-FIT, Adidas's CoolMax or Reebok's Playdry, which wicks (draws) moisture away from your skin and keeps you dry.

Middle layer Only necessary if it's really freezing – try wearing a fleece.

Outer layer Protects you from the elements. Try jackets with taped seams in breathable fabrics such as GORE-TEX.

IIII▶ Hands Thin gloves made from wicking fabrics or cotton will keep your fingers toasty.

IIII▶ Legs Your legs are very effective at generating their own heat, which means a single layer is usually adequate, but double up if you need to. Again, look for snug-fitting bottoms made from wicking fabrics.

IIII▶ Head You lose vast amounts of heat from your head, so keep it covered with a hat.

51 Watch it!

'There are lots of fancy watches out there,' says Sean Falconer, deputy editor of South African *Runner's World*, 'but if you're a beginner, steer clear of any that demand an engineering degree to operate them. All you really need is a stopwatch feature. Another useful feature is a lap counter, which enables you to see how fast you've run every lap, mile or kilometre.' You'll be using your watch on the move, so look out for buttons that are large enough to press easily and big numbers that are easy to see at a glance. Watches that light up in the dark are also very useful on night-time runs.

technique

52

How to burn fat

All kinds of running burn serious calories and fat, which makes it one of the very best exercises for helping you lose weight. However, harder, higher-intensity running will help you burn more fat than easier, lower-intensity running, says top sports nutritionist Anita Bean. 'This is because it burns more calories overall per session,' she says, 'and the more calories you burn, the more fat you break down. It also keeps your metabolism speeded up for longer after you've finished, so you carry on burning calories and fat even when you're back home.' Don't panic if you think you can't do high-intensity running, though – what feels like an easy jog to one person might be high intensity to another. It's all about setting your own personal levels, and finding what represents easy and difficult sessions for you (for more on this, see tip 59). Just make sure you mix in those harder sessions with easier ones so that you stay safe and injury free and don't get discouraged – remember that every single run, whether it's fast or slow, is a massive step along the road towards a leaner, fitter, healthier you. The key thing is to get out there and enjoy yourself.

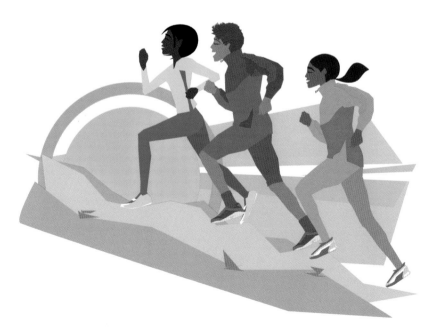

53 Warm up well

When you're embarking on a run, don't just tear out of the front door and run off at full pelt towards the local park. According to sports physiotherapist Georgie Gladwyn, at PhysioCentral in London, the best way to warm up and prepare your body for your run is to do 5 minutes of very gentle jogging that will warm your muscles and get the blood flowing. Then stop for 5 minutes and do the four key lower-body stretches below.

Although recent research has now disputed that stretching before starting to exercise helps prevent you from getting injured, most physios still think it's sensible to take warmed-up muscles through their full range of movement before a run. 'Hold each of these four key stretches for 40 seconds on each leg,' says Gladwyn. Make sure you also hold nice and still in each stretch rather than allowing yourself to bounce, and never stretch so far that it becomes painful.

|||▶ 1. Upper-calf stretch
Push against a wall, tree, fence or lamp-post, with your left leg slightly bent and your right leg extended straight out behind you. Keep both heels flat on the ground and both feet facing forwards. Lean forwards a little, keeping your back straight, and feel the stretch in your upper right calf.

|||▶ 2. Lower-calf stretch Start in the same position as for the upper-calf stretch described above, but now bring your right leg in a little and bend it, lowering your hips slightly and keeping your right heel down. This stretch won't feel as dramatic or as satisfying as the upper-calf stretch, but you should feel it in your Achilles-tendon area.

|||▶ 3. Hamstring (back of thigh) stretch Stand facing a low step or bench and, with your left leg slightly bent and your right leg straight, place your right heel on it. Now bend forwards from the hip,

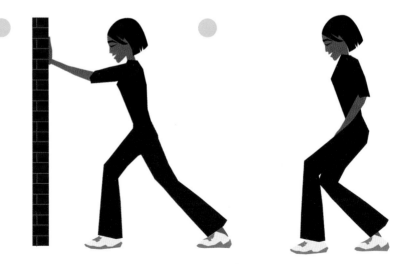

keeping your back straight and sticking your bottom out behind you, so you feel a stretch down the back of your right thigh. Don't round your shoulders, and keep your left leg slightly bent.

IIII▶ **4. Quadriceps (front of thigh) stretch** Stand, holding on to something for support if you need to, and bend your left leg back, taking hold of your left foot with your left hand and easing it in towards your bottom. Keep your right leg slightly bent, and both knees close together – don't let your left knee wander off out to the side or backwards. You should feel a stretch down the front of your left thigh. If you want to increase this stretch, squeeze your buttocks together.

Unless you're feeling very tense in your upper body, you're now ready to set off on your run. Enjoy! If, however, you know you're tight up top, try these three optional extra upper-body stretches, holding each of them for 40 seconds.

IIII▶ **Chest stretch** Clasp your hands together behind your lower back and, pulling your shoulder blades back towards each other, raise your arms slightly to open up your chest.

IIII▶ **Upper-back stretch** Clasp your hands together in front of your chest, palms facing away from your body, and push them away from your chest to feel a lovely stretch opening right up between your shoulder blades.

IIII▶ **Shoulder stretch** Slightly bend your right arm and extend it across your chest, then, placing your left hand on your right upper arm, gently ease your right arm in towards you. Feel the stretch across the back of your right shoulder, then repeat with your left arm. These are also really great stretches to do at work if you're feeling stressed out.

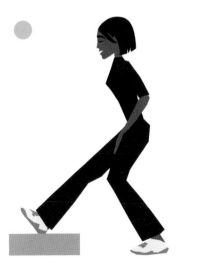

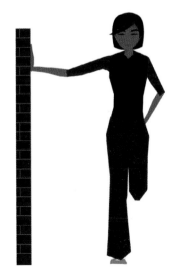

54 Wonderful warm-downs

'Ideally, you don't want to go straight from running flat out to a dead standstill,' says sports physiotherapist Georgie Gladwyn. 'Try to slow down into a walk for the last few minutes of your run, then repeat the four essential stretches in tip 53 (upper calf, lower calf, hamstrings and quads), and add in just one more, the gluteal stretch (shown below), to stop your bottom from feeling sore the day after!' This time, hold each stretch for 40 seconds on each leg and then repeat once more on each side.

Gluteal (bottom) stretch Lying on your back with your knees bent, take your left leg across your right, so your left ankle rests just above your right knee and your left knee points out to the side. Gently draw your right leg in towards you with your hands, so it carries your left leg with it. Keep your left knee turned out to the side, and feel the stretch in your bottom and outer thigh of your left leg (see below).

If you're pushed for time, you can get away with doing just these five basic lower-body stretches. But if you have a bit more time and want to get even more flexible, add these three optional extras...

Inner-thigh stretch Stand with both feet facing forwards and your legs wide apart. Bend your left knee and keep your right leg straight out to the side to feel a stretch right down the inside of your right thigh.

Front-of-hip stretch Kneel with your left knee on the floor, and your right knee bent at a right angle in front of you, keeping your right foot flat on the floor. Now lean your torso gradually forwards, resting your hands on your right leg, until you can feel the stretch in the front of your left hip.

Iliotibial-band stretch To stretch your iliotibial band (a tough band of connective tissue that runs the length of your outer thigh), repeat the front-of-hip stretch as above, but at the same time as leaning forwards, also stick your left hip out to the side a little so you can feel the stretch at the side of your left hip and down the outside of your left thigh, too. If you're feeling really keen, you can also repeat the three upper-body stretches from tip 53.

55 Try a treadmill

It's a great idea for anyone who belongs to a gym to mix sessions on the treadmill with running outdoors, especially in the winter when the weather is bleak! Treadmills are handy as they have a display that allows you to track exactly how fast and how far you're running, and they're also soft on your knees and other joints. To build up your confidence, always start the machine up slowly and raise your speed gradually. Try to avoid holding on to the handrails when you're moving – if you're feeling insecure, you simply need to reduce your speed a little. And experiment with setting the treadmill at a 1% to 2% uphill slope to mimic what it's like to run outdoors.

56 Massage made easy

'If you're injury-prone, rub your calves with some oil before your run,' says Tim Hutchings, running consultant to Reebok. 'It brings blood to the area and starts to loosen things up.'

57 Be style conscious

Everyone has their very own unique running style and you shouldn't try to change yours too much without having an expert watch and advise you. There are, however, some general tips you can follow that should help you get the most out of every run you do, says Graham Anderson, a sports physio at Balance Performance Physiotherapy in London. 'Use whichever tips feel natural from the list to the right,' he says, 'and forget those that feel unnatural – that's

probably a sign that they're wrong for you. Plus, if you do have any problems that keep troubling you, go and get yourself checked out by a running coach or physiotherapist.'

▶ Don't hold your head too far back or forwards – to keep it in the right spot, imagine you're trying to keep a bean bag balanced on top of it.

▶ Keep your eyes looking ahead not down, and your face and jaw relaxed.

▶ Your whole body should be upright, leaning neither forwards nor back, and your shoulders should stay relaxed. Don't let them hunch up.

▶ Aim to let your arms relax and stay close to your body, though you'll find they naturally lift a little higher as you try to run faster or uphill.

▶ Keep your hands loose and never clench them into fists as this can send tension snaking up your arms and into your shoulders. Instead, imagine holding something delicate between your thumb and forefinger.

▶ Push your hips forwards and keep your bottom tucked in rather than stuck out as you run. To get the right position, imagine you're facing a wall and trying to get your hips to touch it. At all costs, avoid running as if you're sitting in a bucket.

▶ Don't try to lift your knees too high unless sprinting. Think instead about driving each knee forwards, not upwards, with each stride.

58 Brilliant bows

Tie your laces in a double bow before every run to stop them coming undone when you're up and running. Having to stop mid run or, worse still, mid-race, to tie a trailing lace is just so annoying.

59 Six successful running sessions

One of the brilliant things about running is that it can be whatever you want it to be – easy or hard, fast or slow, competitive or fun. If running at the same speed over the same distance every time you go out is what suits you, that's great, and you're certainly not doing anything wrong. If, on the other hand, this leaves you feeling a little bored, then there are all sorts of different running sessions you might want to try in order to burn more calories, boost your fitness, get you ready for a race, or simply keep you feeling motivated, challenged and raring to go. We asked Joe Dunbar, sports scientist and running consultant to Nike, to help us put together this list of six super-successful sessions for you to try for size. Use them to keep your running feeling varied, but don't suddenly start doing back-to-back hard sessions – always follow every day of hard work with either a rest day or a day of easier running, so you give your body enough time to recover properly.

Base running

(aka Sunday-morning running)
Perfect for those lazy Sunday mornings, this is the most basic level of running. On a scale of 1 to 10, with 1 being least effort and 10 being toughest, it's sitting pretty in the middle at number 5. Pad along like this and you'll be quite capable of holding a conversation, and checking out what's going on around you. 'This is the kind of speed you'd use if you were going on a longer run, or as an easy recovery run if you'd worked harder the day before,' says Dunbar. The point of it is to build a good base level of fitness, and get your muscles accustomed to taking up and using oxygen and burning fat as fuel.

Steady-state running

(aka running-late-for-Sunday-dinner pace)
This is one step on from base running – the kind of pace you'd go at if you knew you were running a touch late for that Sunday dinner with the in-laws. Although you still feel relaxed and leisurely, and you can still chat away quite well, your effort level has gone up to 7 on the scale. Learn to use this pace on some of your medium-to-long runs and 'It'll get you into a bit better condition, and also start to work your heart and lungs a little harder,' says Dunbar.

Fartlek running

(aka fun-and-frisky running)
This one's fun, fun, fun – honest! Its risqué-sounding name is in fact a Swedish word meaning speed play, and this session asks you to do just that – to play with your speed so you have fun at a variety of different paces. Your session could go a little like this: during a jaunt round the park, you might warm up, run slowly up a small hill, then put in a fast sprint down the other side (as if you'd spotted the last pair of size 6 shoes in the January sales), slow down again until you get

to the next lamp-post or tree, then run fast over gently undulating ground for a minute or two, enjoying the sense of rhythm. Consequently, your effort levels will also vary – from 8 or 9 when you're running fast, back down to 5 as you recover. 'Fartlek is a means of getting your body used to running and working at different speeds,' says Dunbar. 'It's a great way to have your first go at running faster because it's so unstructured – you can simply do what you feel capable of. Think of it as the come-and-have-a-go session.' You can make it feel even more fun by doing it with friends, but do be warned: if you're attempting to do it in the street, you may look a lot less dignified than those base-level Sunday runners!

Tempo running

(aka gets-you-gasping running)
If we're honest, you might not exactly look forward to this type of session, but it's great if you want to bring your running on in leaps and bounds. That's why it's probably best if you do it once you're starting to feel fitter rather than in your first week of entering into the wonderful world of running. On a tempo run your effort level has gone up to 8, you're now breathing hard, and your chat has been left behind as you can only just manage to squeeze out a few words when you're running like this. Which means it actually feels pretty tough. So why bother to put yourself through all this? Because it's a brilliant way to burn calories, work your heart and lungs, and boost

your fitness without having to run for hours on end. 'Run like this and you'll be getting the very best aerobic workout,' says Dunbar. 'And, although it sounds like hard work, it's actually great for lazy runners as you don't have to go on for very long, and you can even take a break in the middle of the session!' Try it yourself by starting with a 5-minute warm-up, then doing 5 minutes of tempo running, taking a 2-minute jog break (during which time you allow your breathing and heart rate to slow a little to prepare for the next effort), then tempo running for another 5 minutes. A great workout in under 20 minutes, and you'll still have time to get to the pub before last orders.

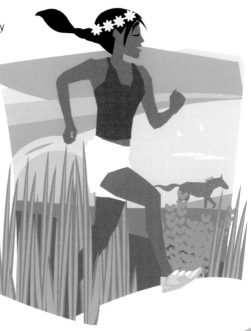

Interval training

(aka quick-slow running)

For interval training you need a bit more inner grit and discipline, and a watch that measures seconds. What you do is alternate between timed bursts of hard running (at an effort level of 8 to 9) and timed easier 'recovery' periods (at an effort level of 2 to 4), which allow you to slow down and get your breath back. 'For your first session, try running hard for 60 seconds, then recovering at a slower pace for 60 seconds, and building up to being able to repeat this pattern eight times,' says Dunbar. The idea is to keep going at the same pace during each of your hard efforts, rather than gradually tailing off. If you find this all too hard, you can do an easier version of intervals where you work slightly less intensely in the hard effort each time (say at an effort level of 7 to 8). Again, sessions like these are great calorie burners and train your body to be able to run faster for longer periods. So when you go back to doing your normal runs, you may find yourself flying along!

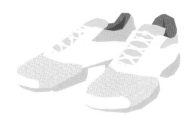

Hill running

(aka 'I-will-survive' running)

Powerful and potent for your body and mind, hill running will improve your mental muscle as well as the muscles in your legs and bottom. Can you go for that promotion? You bet. Dare you ask for that pay rise? Oh yes. Once you can take on that dreaded hill, facing up to just about anything else seems easy. 'Start out gradually with just a couple of bursts of hill running, and work up to doing eight or ten,' says Dunbar. 'Run up the hill for 20 to 30 seconds, gently jog or walk down again, then go up again, repeating the whole process eight times.' You'll also find your effort levels vary just like when you're doing intervals – between 8 to 9 on the way up the hill and between two and four on the way down again. You can choose anything from gentle to steep hills, depending on how hard on yourself you want to make it.

So, what's the point? Having to work against the upward slope of the hill challenges your body in a new way, forcing it to work harder, and it really tests your quad muscles at the front of your thighs. Doing hills will also make you feel pretty invincible. Worth trying for the mental boost alone.

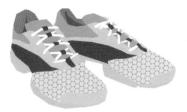

60

Joint effort

If you're worried that running is giving your joints a battering, take heart from the very positive results of an ongoing study at Stanford University, California, USA. From tracking 538 runners and 423 non-runners, all now aged about 58, the study has revealed that the runners developed disabling joint changes an average of 12 years later than the non-runners. In the latest report from the study, only 5% of the runners had developed disabling pain and stiffness, compared with 20% of the non-exercisers.

61

Trick yourself

'Lots of people have a mental block about increasing the distance that they run. If you're finding it tough, try this crafty trick,' says David Francis, 42, a fitness instructor from Oxfordshire. 'Run as far as you can comfortably go on one outing, then the next time you go out, run just one lamp-post or tree farther. It's a really easy way to increase your stamina without it feeling like a struggle.'

62

Beat jelly belly

You might think having strong legs is all that counts in running, but in fact the state of your stomach and back is pretty important, too. If they're weak, they'll tend to sag and curve as you get tired, so your body forms a sort of C-shape, making it much harder for your legs to do their work because they won't have a stable, solid platform to work from. If, however, you have a strong torso, it provides vital support for your whole body and a strong base for your legs to power from, helping you keep on running well even when you're tired.

To develop the right muscles, you need to do core-stability work (so called because it builds a strong and stable core for your whole body). Ideally, try attending Pilates classes, which work on activating not just the superficial muscles of your torso, but also the deeper ones such as the transverse abdominis, which wraps round your whole torso helping keep everything in the right place. 'And when you're out running (and simply day to day), think about tensing and engaging your stomach muscles, and drawing your tummy button towards your spine to help improve your posture and strengthen your torso,' says personal trainer Laura Williams.

63 Rest when you're ill

Don't struggle out for a run when you're feeling awful, especially if you've got a fever, as this could increase your risk of dehydration, heatstroke and even heart failure, says cardio expert Dr Dorian Dugmore of Wellness International at Adidas. 'Your body needs to reserve its energy for fighting off the infection,' he says, 'so don't stress it out by exercising – wait until you're fully recovered before going running again.' It's also a bad idea to run if you've had diarrhoea or been vomiting, once again because you'll be dehydrated.

If you haven't got a temperature but you're feeling ill, use the Neck-Check Method to determine whether you should run – if your symptoms are above the neck (watery eyes, stuffy nose, or a case of the sniffles), you can try running, but reduce the intensity of your session by a third (in other words, treat it as a maintenance session rather than training). If they're below the neck (coughing, chills, muscle aches and nausea), it's best to put your feet up and rest.

64 Shake up your routine

If you always stick to the same running routine, your body will get used to what you're asking it to do, and your fitness level will hit a plateau. Instead, you need to keep on setting yourself new challenges so you keep getting fitter and keep looking better and better! Try the different training plans in Chapter Eight and see tip 70.

65 How to treat an injury

If you've picked up a sprain or a strain, use the acronym RICE to remember what you need to do.

- **R is for rest** Don't attempt to run when you're in pain – you may make things worse.
- **I is for ice** Wrap some crushed ice, or a packet of frozen peas, in a damp tea towel and hold it against the area for no more than 10 minutes every hour. Don't exceed this or you risk frostbite!
- **C is for compression** Quickly put on a compression bandage to stop blood flowing to the area and causing painful swelling and inflammation.
- **E is for elevation** Keep the injured area elevated above the level of your heart to decrease blood flow.

If the pain continues, make sure you see a physiotherapist – don't just keep running with the injury and hoping for the best.

66 Get on track

Find a local running track and try running some laps. If you were sporty at school, it'll bring the excitement of sports day flooding back to you! If you weren't, it'll allow you to rewrite history by proving just how fit and fab you are right now.

67 Count off the miles

This tip is from the marathon ace Paula Radcliffe herself. When the going gets tough in a race, she counts slowly to 300 in her head. By the time she's got there, she's run a mile and it's time to start all over again. A word of warning – expect to make it to more like 600 if you're trying it – Paula runs about five-minute miles during a marathon!

The beginner's version? 'I'm just starting out,' says novice runner Kate Monkhouse, 29, director of the London Civic Forum, 'so I run for 100 paces, then walk for 50, and keep going like that. I find counting is a really good way to stop me worrying about how I'm doing, and keeps my head feeling clear.'

68 Get vain

Always bag the treadmill facing the mirror. This gives you a fantastic opportunity to focus on your posture and running technique, spot and correct anything you're doing wrong and, of course, ponder whether your new pink running top really clashes with the colour your face goes when you're a bit sweaty.

69 Take it steady

Don't expect to increase both your speed and your distance at once. Choose a shorter distance if you want to try going faster, and if you want to try going farther, slow down your pace. Plus, make sure you follow hard days with easier runs so you don't put too much strain on your body. 'Don't let anyone push you too hard,' says Jennie Francis, 45, a hypnotherapist from London. 'The first time I started running, the trainer at my gym encouraged me to go too fast too soon, and I ended up with shin splints. I think it was because I look quite sporty and have big, muscular legs, so people tend to try and push me! The second time I tried running, I took it at my own pace, did what felt right, and fared much better.'

70 Spice up your workouts

A great way to add interest to your running programme and get even fitter is to try cross-training. This simply means throwing different kinds of workouts into the mix to help you develop new physical and mental skills. 'If you're a regular runner, I'd recommend you also try cycling and aqua-jogging (in a pool wearing a flotation belt or vest) to improve leg endurance while minimising impact,' says US fitness expert Martica Heaner. 'Also, try swimming for all-over body conditioning, martial arts for their mind, body and postural benefits, weights workouts for strength, and stretching to keep you supple.'

71 How to stay injury-free

||||▶ Always wear good trainers and replace them every 600 miles or so.

||||▶ Warm up and stretch – while it can't prevent injury, it's a good idea to take your muscles and joints through a full range of movement before you start a run (see tip 53).

||||▶ Vary the surfaces you run on to reduce impact on your joints – try to run on grass, trails and a track as well as roads and pavements.

||||▶ Be aware of any areas in your body that are tensing up while you're running and consciously try to relax them.

||||▶ Get any niggling problems seen to early by a qualified physiotherapist – neglecting aches and pains can put stress on other areas of your body.

||||▶ Don't try to take things too fast too soon and always have a rest day after a hard session.

72 Six-packs for speed

Not convinced speed-training's worth the effort? Think again. 'When I was at university,' says Loren Jackson, 34, a lawyer from Durban, South Africa, 'my running club challenged any runners who hadn't previously done speed-training to try doing it once a week for a month. Anyone whose performance in a 5K (3-mile) race didn't improve as a result was promised a six-pack of

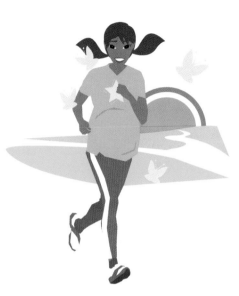

beer. As far as I know, no one ever won the beer!'

73 Can you run when pregnant?

It's certainly not the time to take up running if you've never run before, but if you're fit, healthy and used to running, there's no reason why you can't keep going gently. You will need to make a few changes though, as it's important not to get totally breathless, and not to get too hot and sweaty while you're exercising. If you take the intensity of your runs down a notch and listen to what feels right for your body, then you should be able to continue enjoying your running while pregnant. Paula Radcliffe showed the way for lots of women when she took part in a 10K race – at a more gentle pace than her normal blistering one – when just over five months pregnant. Once you've given birth, speak to your GP about how

soon you can start running again.
If you've not had a Caesarean or any
other major complications, many
doctors will tell you it's fine to run
about six weeks after the birth. But
again, base your decision on how your
body is feeling.

74 Put your feet up

Here's one piece of
expert advice we know
you're going to love: to get fit it's just
as important to rest as it is to run.
'When you run,' says Rob Spedding,
assistant editor at British *Runner's
World*, 'your muscles and ligaments
develop microscopic tears and you use
up your energy resources. This isn't a
problem if you give them time to repair
themselves by resting. However, if you
don't give yourself time off, these tiny
tears can become full-on strains, the
used-up energy can lead to fatigue and
your running can suffer massively. Rest
is especially important after hard
races, long runs and speed work.'

The easiest way to make sure you
get enough rest is to pencil into your
schedule at least one day off a week
when you take it really easy and don't
do any kind of workout. Beginners
should take more time off, as should
older runners. Spedding also suggests
you nominate one month each year as
a rest month. 'Cut your overall mileage
in half,' he says, 'and replace some of
your runs with cross-training activities.
It's a great way to recharge your
batteries and keep your enthusiasm for
running topped up.'

75 Perform the Rope Trick

If you
think hills are hellish,
try this tip used by Bruce Fordyce, the
legendary South African runner who
won the unbelievably hilly Comrades
ultra-marathon an amazing nine times.
'When you're tackling a hill,' he says,
'imagine you're pulling yourself up it
using two parallel ropes. Really power
your arms but keep your hands nice
and relaxed. It truly does help turn
mountains into molehills.'

76 Get enough sleep

'As you start
running more, you'll
probably also find you need to start
sleeping for longer periods,' says
Professor Tim Noakes, Discovery health
professor of exercise and sports
science at the University of Cape
Town, South Africa. 'If, for example,
you run for two hours, you may well
need an extra hour's sleep as well,
which means you'll have to learn how
to budget your time to fit in the
running and extra sleeping.'

motivation

77 Get fancy!

Want to feel like a film star for a few hours? Fancy having crowds straining to get a glimpse of you, hearing wild cheers when you finally make your appearance, and having photographers leaping out at every bend in the road? All you have to do is enter any well-supported race, slip into a fancy-dress outfit and *voilà*! Eat your heart out, Nicole Kidman! 'Dressing up can be tremendously motivating,' says top life coach Fiona Harrold, 'as you'll get twice as much support from the crowd, who'll really appreciate the effort you went to.' One word of warning, though: take your outfit on a few trial runs before race day or you may find your Batman cape hampers rather than hastens your progress.

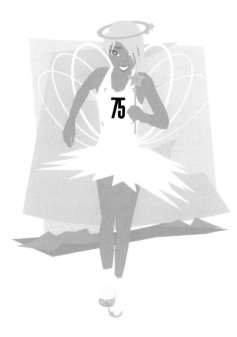

78 Fib to yourself

'I have the running bug and no kind of medicine can make it go away,' says Stuart Major, 41, a policeman from Surrey. 'And yet, like most runners I know, there are times when I really don't feel like going for a run. I get home from work, I'm tired and hungry, and all I want to do is sit and watch TV. On those days I tell myself to do just 20 to 30 minutes – I'll be back before I know it. So I head out and, after ten minutes, I usually feel much better and consider running 40 or 50 minutes. When I've finished the run, I no longer feel tired or hungry and am thrilled I managed to do it.'

79 Turn the postie into your personal trainer

One of the best ways to feel like a 'real' runner is to subscribe to a health and fitness magazine such as *Zest*, or a running magazine such as *Runner's World*. Each time a new issue lands with a thump on your doormat, you'll be reminded that you're a runner, a runner who's committed enough (even if you've only been running for a couple of weeks) to invest in a year's subscription. Magazines are bursting with the latest fitness news, tips and inspirational stories, and *Runner's World* contains listings of races near you. When you're feeling demotivated, a quick read may be all it takes to reinspire and encourage you.

80 Go running somewhere spectacular

Few things are as mood-boosting as running in an amazing location. Choose one of these suggestions and feel your spirits soar...

⭐ **Run beside a river, lake or ocean** if you want to feel soothed and calmed. Even better if it's warm enough for you to take a dip in afterwards.

⭐ **Run somewhere famous.** Any place that starred in a film will do. Try scooting up the steps of the Philadelphia Museum of Art and you'll be treading in the footsteps of Sly Stallone in the *Rocky* movies; run along Scotland's West Sands beach with distant views of the steeple-studded skyline of St Andrews, and you'll be recreating the legendary scene in *Chariots of Fire*

(don't forget to hum the Vangelis theme tune!); run along a straight highway and you can pretend you're starring in a scene from *Forrest Gump* (chanting 'Run, Forrest, run' to yourself is optional!).

⭐ **Run in a foreign capital city.** Invariably they're glamorous and packed with legendary, amazing landmarks. Running – especially along famous marathon routes like the River Seine towards the Eiffel Tower or down swanky Fifth Avenue in New York – beats taking a tour bus or taxi every time, and means you'll gain an infinitely better understanding of the city's layout and see things you'd otherwise have missed.

⭐ **Run anywhere hilly or high.** You might struggle to climb to the top but the views when you get there will be so awesome they'll make you feel on top of the world.

81 Train your brain

'There are certain things runners should never, ever utter,' says Frank Horwill, coach to 43 international runners. 'One of them is, "I can't." Instead, say, "I will try." Exercise your willpower by doing more of what you most dislike in training and racing (or whatever you know is a weakness, such as hills or speed-training). Start small and gradually progress from there.'

82 Run for charity

Raising money for charity can be a tremendous motivator when you're flagging in a race (or tempted to skip a training session). For the past five years, Dale Brumfield, 44, a medical insurance broker from Richmond, USA, has participated in the Relay For Life, an event that raises money for cancer research. Each year he has run for up to 20 hours at a stretch, and in so doing has raised close to $10,000 (about £6,300). Why does he do it? 'A burning desire to find a cure for cancer keeps me circling the track for all those hours,' he says. 'I've lost too many friends and family members to cancer. And when compared with enduring the wretched sickness of chemotherapy and radiation, running 260-plus laps round a track seems like the least I can do. If someone can survive cancer and cancer treatment, I figure I can survive a 104km (65-mile) run.'

83 Put fun first

'Fun should be your ultimate goal in every run or race you do – that way, you're 1,000% more likely to stick to a running plan – for the long haul!' says personal trainer Jane Forbes. Run past interesting shops, chat to fellow runners, indulge in carb-rich jellybeans – whatever makes you smile, just do it! 'Avoid grimacing, look ahead instead of down, and greet other runners with a cheery "Hi!"' says Peter Grecian, 40, a computer special-effects expert from Kingston-upon-Thames. 'I also believe that the time spent running should be influenced by the weather forecast and chance of experiencing a spectacular sunset, rather than guilt-inspired, grim determination.'

84 Be a show-off!

You've run that 5K (3 miles), you've made it through a 10K (6-mile) race, you've conquered that marathon – now revel in your success and use it to inspire you to even greater efforts. Hang your medals where you can easily see them, compile a running album (include your race numbers, certificates, photos and newspaper cuttings showing your finishing times) or frame a photo of you triumphantly crossing the finish line, arms aloft. When you're finding it hard to get motivated, they'll help rekindle your enthusiasm.

85 Reward yourself

Learn to associate running with fun, pleasure and feeling good by giving yourself a reward after each run, with either a healthy treat, or a slightly wicked one. As Karen Harverson, 35, a journalist from Johannesburg, South Africa, says, 'Every Sunday, my husband and I promise ourselves we can pop into a café for an ice-cold can of coke at the 8K mark of our 10K run. I sneakily drag out drinking mine for as long as possible to get my breath back before we tackle the final stretch. I can tell you, coke never tastes as good as it does on Sundays!'

Cathie Greasley, 28, a promotions executive from London, has a similar strategy: 'I tell myself that if I go for a run I can enjoy some of my favourite treats guilt-free,' she says, 'and often have a glass of wine afterwards. Some people say, "What's the point?" but for me that is the whole point!'

Don't forget to congratulate yourself afterwards! Elizabeth Roberts, 29, an academic from Perth, Australia, found this revolutionised her runs. 'When I first started running,' she says, 'I'd really beat myself up if I didn't achieve my goals. I didn't really enjoy running then – I just gritted my teeth and got on with it. I finally broke this destructive cycle one day when, having met my goal, I just said to myself, as an invisible coach might have done, "Well done. You're brilliant!" The change it made in me was remarkable – I felt glowy all over. From then on I've tried to do it at the end of every run. And even if I haven't met my goal, I still try to say something encouraging such as, "You tried hard at that." I actually look forward to my runs now – especially the pep talks I get afterwards.'

86 Beat the toxic ten minutes

Many first-time runners are put off by how terrible they feel in the first ten minutes of a run. 'If I feel this horrible now, it's not going to get any better,' they reason, and promptly give up running for ever. We've been running for years and were amazed when we both confessed to suffering the first ten minutes from hell each time we run. But cross that magic ten-minute barrier and we guarantee you'll be feeling much, much better – trust us, we know! It's simply that your body has to gear itself up and make the transition from being sedentary to running. Harness your willpower, stick it out for just ten minutes and it'll all be easier from there on in.

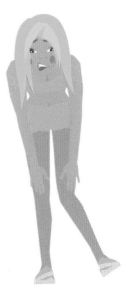

87 Go clubbing!

Running clubs aren't just for blink-and-you'll-miss-'em runners – most welcome beginners with open arms (visit www.runtrackdir.com/ukclubs to find one). Here are just a few reasons why going clubbing may turn out to be the best thing you ever did:

▐▐▐▶ Having to turn up at a set time each week means you'll have a date in your diary and so you'll be more likely to go running that day rather than slink off to the pub after work.

▐▐▐▶ You'll get access to the combined expertise of coaches and other more experienced runners so you'll be able to learn from their mistakes without having to make them yourself. You'll also be encouraged to do speed-training sessions, which you may otherwise be tempted to avoid like athlete's foot if you run solo.

▐▐▐▶ Clubs are highly sociable and often host parties, weekends away and nights out, so you'll gain an instant circle of friends along with a fitter body. You may even meet Mr (or Ms) Right! 'My friend and I trawled virtually all the running clubs in London looking for someone we fancied,' says Caroline Yarnell, 43, a postgraduate student who's now living in Sydney, Australia. 'They usually have a lot more male than female runners so you can take your pick! While training at the running track in Battersea Park, our coach suggested I do something called social sprints with another runner called Tony – we had to sprint to a set point and then walk

back talking to each other. The coach's plan worked – Tony and I got on like a house on fire and have now been married ten years.'

88 Run to take part, not to win

In every race there's only room for three people up on the podium, so don't worry if you're not one of them. Running races is meant to be fun, so unless you answer to the name of Paula Radcliffe, don't obsess about where you're going to come (in some popular races it's not unusual to come 4,899th!). Focus on having a good time rather than achieving a good time. 'When you're lagging behind in a race,' says Catherine Mokwena, 41, an administrator from Johannesburg, South Africa, 'remind yourself that it took a lot of courage just to enter – thousands wouldn't even dream of it – and take inspiration from that.'

89 Disobey your mother…

… and run after the boys! It's a brilliant way for all you girls to improve in leaps and bounds. Men make excellent running partners because they're naturally faster than women, so this will force you to improve in order to keep up. They're also far more competitive than women, which may in turn help bring out your own mean streak. Just don't overdo it, and take rest days after hard runs.

90 Choose your mental mode

You may not be consciously aware of this, but when you're running you'll be in one of two mental states: you'll either be associating (concentrating on how you're running) or dissociating (letting your mind wander). 'When you're a beginner runner, you tend to associate,' says Helen Collins, editor of Australian *Runner's World*. 'You're concerned with progress, with how this new exciting activity feels, and are conscious of your heart rate and breathing, and having thoughts like, "Oh, this hill goes on for ever." But when you get to that level of fitness where you can cruise comfortably, you tend to dissociate. Your mind starts to follow fairly complicated trains of thought and the kilometres clock by without you noticing. You no longer have to think about the effort required as relaxed running has become effortless.'

However, it's also possible to choose consciously which mode to run in – here are some tips on which one to go for and when…

Choose association if… you want running to be an escape from your everyday problems. Want 20 minutes of not fretting about that blazing row you had with your boyfriend? Try associating. It's also a great way to run with better posture as you'll be monitoring your body constantly (try working from your head down and checking each body part in turn – head lifted? Yes. Shoulders relaxed? Yes. Hands unclenched? Yes. See our posture pointers in tip 57 for more on what to aim for).

Association is also useful if you want to run faster. According to researchers at the University of Cape Town, South African, runners who were encouraged to monitor their body signals were inspired to run harder. In shorter races, says Collins, you're likely to find yourself associating as you'll be constantly monitoring your performance to assess if you need to slow down or increase your pace, how close you are to reaching the finish line and where you are in the field.

Choose dissociation if… you find that concentrating on running makes your mileage creep by at a snail's pace and you want to be distracted from how far you still need to go. It's also handy if you need head space to work through problems. 'The act of running can work almost like meditation,' says Collins, 'calming your mind and allowing anxiety, anger and frustration to dissipate.' Dissociation is particularly useful in longer races, when you can switch between keeping track of your performance (association) and allowing yourself to think about whatever takes your fancy (whether that's last night's TV, what you're going to have for dinner or the scenery you're passing through). 'While this strategy probably won't help you run your best time,' says Collins, 'it can help you get through the race more easily and with more enjoyment.'

91 Navigate your neighbourhood

Beware of boredom! Running the same old route week in, week out, is guaranteed to make you feel like a rat on a treadmill (and won't pose any new challenges for your muscles). Instead, photocopy a map of your neighbourhood and go exploring. Use a highlighter pen to colour in all the roads you've run on during each session, aiming to colour them all in eventually. Or try this tip from Helen Terry, 34, a teacher from Newcastle-under-Lyme. 'When it's dark by 4pm in winter and it would be so much easier to hit the sofa with a large gin and tonic,' she says, 'I try to plan routes round the streets with the most outrageous Christmas lights. They make me smile when I whizz by in the car, so a chance to pass them slowly and really take them in is a bonus that helps inspire me to run!'

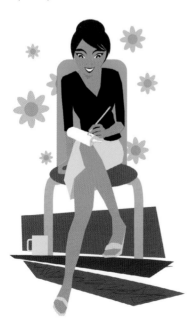

92 Use your imagination

Your mind, not your leg muscles, is the single most important thing that will get you round in a race or on a run (or past of your front door). Try these mental tricks for size:

▐▐▐➤ 'When I'm running on the treadmill, I usually listen to music by a singer I can visualise,' says Nishel Priya, 25, a sales consultant from London. 'My favourites are Christina Aguilera, J-Lo and Kylie. They all have great bodies and when I picture them while I'm running, it helps motivate me, as I aspire to look as good as they do.'

▐▐▐➤ 'Whenever I need a bit of help getting out of the door,' says Julie Brown, 23, a PA from New York, 'I imagine the sensation of the wind in my hair, of sun on my face and the smell of the grass crushed underfoot. It's usually enough to make me want to rush outside and run.'

▐▐▐➤ 'To keep myself amused while I run, I speculate about the lives of the people who live in the houses I'm running past,' says Janet Watson, 36, an economics teacher from Sydney, Australia. 'I imagine what they look like, where they work, and how they've decorated their homes. I escape to this fantasy world and before I know it, I'm back at my own front door.'

93 Find your best time of day

Some experts say the best time of day to train is in the evening, when your body's had a chance to warm up during the day and your joints and muscles are at their most flexible. However, if you're always knackered or ravenous (or often work late or have childcare commitments) then that's not going to be the best slot for you. Neither is going out at 6.30am if getting up is always the most horrendous, gut-wrenching five minutes of your day. Be nice to yourself and never make yourself do something you don't want to do (at least not to start with!). Remember you want to enjoy running. 'When I first took up running,' says Emily Thorne, 27, a beautician from Edinburgh, 'I promised myself that I would never make myself run at weekends (they were sacred) or before or after work (when I'd feel too tired), so I always went out at lunchtime during the week. However, as I started enjoying running more, I renegotiated my terms with myself as I wanted to go on longer runs. Now I quite happily run at weekends or after work – but never before work as I'm like a grizzly bear with a sore head in the morning!'

⭐ **Go for mornings if**… you want to get a buzz (and a metabolism boost) that lasts all day, or if you're a morning person and you want to get it done before anything else can distract you (no one's going to ask you whether you can work late or come out for drinks before work, are they?).

⭐ **Go for lunchtimes if**… other commitments mean it's the only hour in the day you have solely for you, if you want to save money as you'd only go out shopping or eat loads if you didn't, or if you want to maximise your chances of seeing some sunshine.

⭐ **Go for evenings if**… you want to use running as a form of stress relief, you want to run without any time constraints or you want to incorporate your run into your commute home.

⭐ **Go for any window of opportunity if**… your schedule is unpredictable or you have a hectic social life. Meeting friends for a drink? Tell them you'll be 45 minutes late and have a quick dash around the park first. Going to a concert? Change into your running gear in the loos afterwards and run to the station instead of getting a cab (yes, it has been known!).

94 Practise negative thinking

If you hate being told what to do (and see a running programme as a kind of strict headmistress who's bossing you around), pander to your rebellious streak by telling yourself you will never ever run when you don't feel like it – but add the proviso that you must *really, really, really* not feel like it before you can give yourself permission to play hooky. You'll probably only skip a handful of sessions a year – and enjoy the ones you do, as you know you've had the option not to go if you didn't want to.

95 Talk the talk

Talking is a great way to monitor whether you're running at the right pace. If you're running steadily, you should be able to talk quite easily, but if you're doing a tempo session (see tip 59), not being able to talk shows you're putting in a good effort. Don't forget, too, that it's a fantastic way to make a longish run magically feel like a shorter one. Take along a running partner or hitch up with a fellow competitor in a race and get chatting. Aim for at least 10,000 words per mile (!) and you'll be at the finish line (or at your front door) before you know it. Alternatively, sing! Katherine Lee, 25, an office manager from Croydon, does just that. 'The song I sing depends on how fast I'm running,' she says. 'If I'm speeding along, I think happy thoughts and sing chart hits to myself, and if it's a slower run, the more romantic side of me comes out and I opt for a love song.'

Wimpie de Bruyn, 68, from Pretoria, South Africa, has been running for more than 30 years and has kept a diary ever since he started running on 1 January 1973. In it he's recorded everything from the weather to who he ran with – along with exactly how far he ran, both in training and in races. He's now able to boast having run more than 80,000km (50,000 miles), equivalent to running twice round the world! Another South African runner, Frank Clarke, 67, a retired general manager from Durban, hasn't missed a single day's training since 9 August 1977. That's more than 9,600 consecutive days of running (not something we recommend, by the way – see tip 74 for the benefits of rest!). You may not get as far as Wimpie or go out as often as Frank, but you could aim to run across the Atlantic or go running three times a week for the next 20 years...

96 Be a pen pal

We've said it before but your pen really is your biggest ally in helping you to stick with the programme. Use it to slot your training sessions into your diary like Keren Lerner, 28, a website designer from London. 'I make plans to go running with a friend,' she says, 'and diarise it as I would any other appointment.' Keeping a running diary is an amazing motivational tool as it'll help you keep tabs on your progress and give you clues as to what does and doesn't work for you. To get you started, we've put together a six-month running diary for you to use at the back of this book – see pages 206–21.

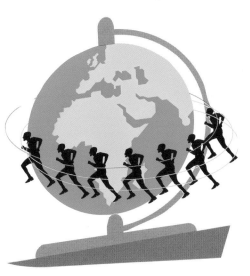

97 Enter a race

Don't be intimidated by races as they can give you a massive motivation boost. They're a brilliant way of providing you with a goal, meeting other runners and assessing your progress. Plus, they're the ultimate way to make sure you stick to your training programme – the mere thought of struggling through a race because you haven't trained can be enough to spur you on to run regularly. Sharon Lindores, 35, a journalist, found this out when she moved to Edmonton in Canada, where winters are so harsh that some runners put nails on the bottom of their shoes to get better grip on icy patches! 'I found running in the dark at -40°C (-40°F) really hard,' she says, 'so to keep me motivated, I signed up for a spring race. Running in the winter made me feel as if I was defying the elements and, when spring finally arrived, I was in good-enough shape to do my race and enjoy longer runs in the good weather.'

A race is also a good opportunity to see places you've been dying to visit. Always wanted to zoom round Silverstone Racetrack? Potter along Charles Bridge in Prague? Run through Berlin's Brandenburg Gate? There are races that will allow you to do all these things.

98 Buddy up

Training with a running partner is a sure-fire way to make runs more fun (and frequent!). Emma Simpson, 31, a designer from Sussex, swears by running with a partner, or in her case two. 'I was determined to regain my former fitness after having my baby,' she says, 'so I talked two mums from my antenatal class into coming with me once a week while our partners looked after our children. It's hard to give yourself permission to have time off when you're a parent, but going for a run with my friends gives us time away from our partners and children and a chance to have a laugh and a natter while relaxing and getting fit.'

99 Be competitive

Competition can add a whole new sense of excitement to your running, says Bud Baldaro, running consultant with Adidas, 'as long as you don't get too carried away or let it make you feel panicked or pressured. Start out being competitive with yourself – set yourself a realistic challenge that demands a certain degree of effort, such as doing a 5K (3-mile) race in under 35 minutes, then see if you can do it faster the next time you run that race. Another way to foster your competitive streak is to assess your improvement by measuring yourself against other runners. In a big race, for example, in which you came in the top 2,000 one year, you could aim to come in the top 1,500 the next year. Continually setting yourself targets and reaching them will make you feel fantastic.'

100 One potato, two potato

Losing weight can be a marvellous incentive to keep running. 'Each time you lose a couple of pounds, buy the same weight in potatoes and keep them in a bag in your kitchen,' says Karen Reeve, 28, a director's PA from Somerset. 'Then, when you want to skip a run you're scheduled to do, pick up the bag and say to yourself, "Running helped me lose this much weight – do I really want to miss this session?" Those potatoes will help you realise you'd be better off going running after all.'

101 Just one last thing...

Yes, we know we said 100 tips but we needed room for just one more! If you're feeling mindboggled by all the advice we've just given you, don't forget the most important tip of all. Running is meant to be fun. Don't get hung up on whether you're doing it right or wrong (unless it's injuring or hurting you, of course) – the more you run, the more you'll learn. In the meantime, just get out and enjoy it!

POTATOES

○ ○ ○ Now you're ready to
take the next step and
run that little bit farther,
we've devised three training
plans to speed you along.
Plus we've got info on
cross-training workouts
to boost your running
potential, and the low-down
on how to enjoy every race
to the maximum...

8

get even
better

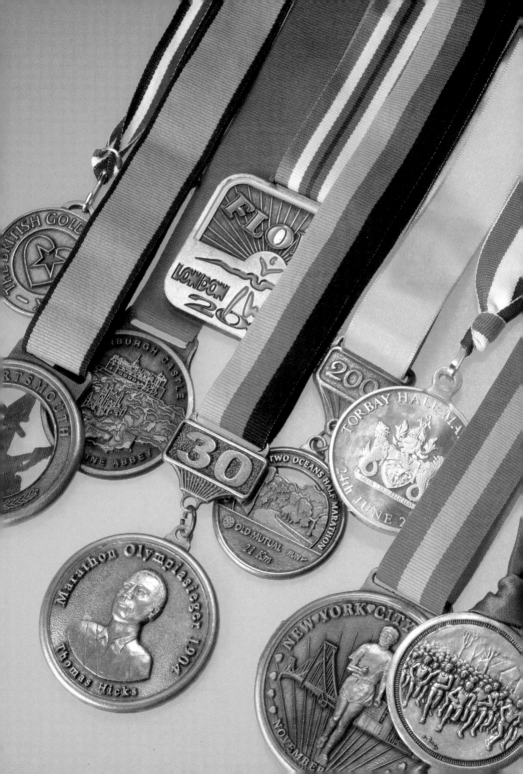

Racing ahead!

Want some excitement in your life? Then enter a race
– you'll never look back...

Falling in love with running is quite like settling into a new relationship – after the initial heart-racing, cheek-flushing thrill has worn off, you have to work hard to avoid slipping into the equivalent of a TV-dinners and slippers-by-the-fire comfort zone, where you stick to what you know, and do the same two laps of the park on the same three nights every week. Of course, there's nothing wrong with getting cosy and comfy with running; it's just that if you dare to challenge yourself and inject a little more

excitement into your running routine, you'll get so much more fun from it. Muster the courage to take on a new challenge and you'll be repaid a hundred times over by the changes you see in not just your body but your mind, your attitude and your whole life.

get faster, go farther
This chapter is dedicated to helping you improve, whether you want to start running faster or go farther. We believe the best way for you to do this is to enter a race so you have a goal to aim

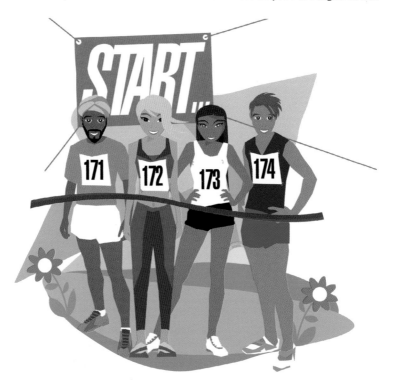

for. If the mere thought of this makes your knees knock with fear, don't worry – we've been there, too, and everyone has to start somewhere. Even the legendarily awesome marathon supremo Paula Radcliffe came 299th (out of 600 plus) in her first national race, and just look at her now!

glory and glamour

There's nothing like the feeling of fear and anticipation as you line up with hundreds of other runners on the start line, or the glory and glamour of running towards the finish line that brings out the natural show-off in us all. To take you smoothly into your first race and beyond, we've put together three training plans that'll help you run any distance you've set your heart

on. If you followed The 60-Second-Secret Plan in Chapter Six, you're already capable of doing a 5K (3-mile) race, so the plans in this chapter will help get you round a 10K (6-mile) race, a half-marathon (21km/13.1 miles) and a marathon (42km/26.2 miles). They're designed for you to work through in sequence, so you build up your fitness gradually, and enjoy every step. Each one follows a slightly different format as each was designed by a different expert, but they all contain principles that will be familiar to you from Chapters Six and Seven, such as walk/run sessions and tempo running. Plus we've got info on which cross-training workouts are best for runners, and tips and advice on how to get the most from them.

Five ways to start improving – right now!

1 Remember where you started. If you think you can't improve, remind yourself of just how far you've already come – and then start imagining how much farther you can go.

2 Get some support. It's hard to improve all alone – run with someone who's better than you, or join a running club to provide extra motivation.

3 Race against the clock. Run with a watch and aim to keep beating your times. Try a two-lap run, on which you time your first lap, then aim to run faster on the second lap.

4 Be kind to yourself. 'Push your limits,' says Lisa Buckingham, 25, a sub-editor from London, 'but never so far that you feel really awful. Your brain stores information like that, and if you start associating running with pain or feeling terrible, your motivation will melt away.'

5 Get inspired. Go along and spectate at the first race you're intending to run. It'll help you get familiar with the course and give you a good idea of what to expect on the day. But best of all, when you see the cheering crowds and how much fun everyone is having, it'll motivate you to join in.

'My most memorable race'

Broken stereos, spa baths and achieving the impossible –
six runners share their favourite race-day memories...

" When my Walkman failed just as the gun went off on the start line of a 5K (3-mile) Race For Life, I was gutted. Listening to music was the only way I'd learnt to run – the beat kept me at an even pace and stopped me panicking as I couldn't hear how out of breath I was! But as people all around me surged forwards, **I realised it was too late to chicken out, even though the last time I'd been in a race I'd been jumping down the school field in a sack**. Those three miles were the hardest I've ever run, but I didn't stop or slow down once. When I finally crossed the finish line, red-faced and panting, I was ecstatic. I love running outside now, and despite the fact that I can easily run more than three miles, that first race was my most important achievement. My medal still reminds me that I can do anything when I put my mind to it.'
Charlotte Stacey, 26, journalist, London

'I'll always be grateful to my first race, the Flora Light Women's Challenge, for teaching me to run outdoors. I'd been running on the treadmill at the gym for a couple of years but was always too shy and embarrassed to run outside. But then I decided to do the race with my friend, and **we just treated it as a laugh, telling each other we could stop whenever we wanted**. I loved it and never looked back – straight after that, I started running on Clapham Common while training for the Flora London Marathon, and running on family weekends away. Now I've got a dog and love going for runs in the woods with her. It's opened up a whole new world!' **Liza Robinson, 38, physiotherapist, Surrey**

'My favourite race is a half-marathon run in Ein Gedi at the Dead Sea, the lowest point on earth. **To your left is the Dead Sea and to your right are the Jordean mountains, creating one of the most picturesque locations in the world**. After the race, you can go to the spa in Ein Gedi and soak in baths rich with salt and other minerals, making this a very relaxing and enjoyable weekend.'
Stewart Granby, 45, accounting manager, Shorashim, Israel

'Running the Adidas Mini London Marathon (4.2km/2.65 miles) was hard but it was the **best day of my life!** I felt I'd really achieved something.'
Leo Kellock, 12, pupil, London

'During my first race (the16K/10-mile Great South Run in Portsmouth), I realised **running is as much about what's going on in your head as what you're doing with your body.** As I got tired in the final stages of the run, I found myself literally saying out loud, "You can do it, you can do it." I got to the finish having run the whole way and just felt so proud that I wanted to cry.'
Maria O'Keefe, 32, hair salon creative director, London

'The most emotional thing I've ever done is the Comrades Marathon, an 89K (55.6-mile) race from Pietermaritzburg to Durban in South Africa. For 16 years I watched the race on TV, from the dawn start to the final gun at dusk, and felt choked with emotion. Then, one year, I found myself shivering on the start line and couldn't hold back the tears. My fondest memory of the whole run was passing a school for handicapped kids. The tots were in calipers, on crutches, or with artificial legs, and those that could had their hands outstretched for us to high five as we ran past.

With 28K (17.5 miles) to go, I thought I wouldn't make it before the cut-off time, but as I got closer to the finish, **all I can recall is the spectators willing us on, eager to help in any way they could**, even if it was just wiping my sunglasses clean on their dry T-shirts. At the entrance to the stadium where the race finished, I started retching but the crowd yelled, "Don't stop!" and a stranger grabbed my wrist and said, "You've got to run! Stay with me."
All I could think as I ran towards the line (and the man who fires the final gun to signal that the cut-off time has been reached and you're not allowed to finish) was, "You can't be sick here in front of the TV cameras!" As I staggered to the finish, the spectators were beside themselves, screaming us in, willing us to make it... and I did, by 18 seconds. A few days after the race, a friend, who avoids all exercise, called me to ask how it went and said, "What took you so long?" **Pam Newby, 54, webmaster, Cape Town, South Africa** 🙷

YOUR 10K PLAN

Who's it good for?

Anyone who has run a 5K (3-mile) race and is ready to go that little bit farther – 10K is equivalent to just over 6 miles. It's a great taster race for new runners, and hip and trendy types, with races like the Run London Nike 10K attracting hordes of 20- and 30-somethings into running for the first time. It is also ideal for speed freaks who'd rather run faster over a shorter distance, and anyone who comes out in a rash at the thought of doing a marathon.

How does it feel? Lovely! It's just far enough to feel like a 'proper' race, and to allow you to test yourself, but without feeling like too much of a hard slog or meaning you have to train too hard.

How long will it take? Less than 45 minutes and you're flying, about an hour is good, over an hour and you'll be in good company with the slightly more leisurely but still perfectly respectable runners.

What's the plan? A ten-week programme designed by sports scientist Joe Dunbar, who's been a running consultant to Nike for many years and designed training plans for the Run London Nike 10K (visit www.runlondon.com).

Effort levels for your sessions are given in brackets, with 1 being the easiest and 10 the hardest.

WEEK ONE

Monday: Walk 20 mins (effort level 2 to 4)
Tuesday: Rest
Wednesday: Run 5 mins (effort level 5), walk 3 mins (effort level 2). Repeat once more (Total: 16 mins)
Thursday: Rest
Friday: Run 7 mins (effort level 5), walk 2 mins (effort level 2). Repeat once more (Total: 18 mins)
Saturday: Rest
Sunday: Run 15 mins (effort level 5)

WEEK TWO

Monday: Walk 30 mins (effort level 2 to 4)
Tuesday: Rest
Wednesday: Run 10 mins (effort level 5), walk 2 mins (effort level 2 to 4). Repeat once more (Total: 24 mins)
Thursday: Rest
Friday: Run 7 mins (effort level 5), walk 2 mins (effort level 2 to 4). Repeat once more (Total: 18 mins)
Saturday: Rest
Sunday: Run 20 mins (effort level 5)

WEEK THREE

Monday: Walk 30 mins (effort level 4)
Tuesday: Rest
Wednesday: Run 15 mins (effort level 6)
Thursday: Rest
Friday: Run 10 mins (effort level 5), walk 3 mins (effort level 4). Repeat once more (Total: 26 mins)
Saturday: Rest
Sunday: Run 25 mins (effort level 5)

WEEK FOUR
Monday: Run 15 mins (effort level 5)
Tuesday: Rest
Wednesday: Run 20 mins
(effort level 5)
Thursday: Rest
Friday: Run 15 mins (effort level 7)
Saturday: Rest
Sunday: Run 30 mins (effort level 5)

WEEK FIVE
Monday: Run 20 mins (effort level 5)
Tuesday: Rest
Wednesday: Run 20 mins
(effort level 7)
Thursday: Rest
Friday: Run 25 mins
(effort level 5 to 6)
Saturday: Rest
Sunday: Run 35 mins (effort level 5)

WEEK SIX
Monday: Walk 40 mins
(effort level 3 to 4)
Tuesday: Rest
Wednesday: Run 5 mins (effort level
5), then repeat the following 5 times:
run 1 min (effort level 8 to 9), walk
1 min (effort level 2) (Total: 15 mins)
Thursday: Rest
Friday: Run 25 mins (effort level 5 to 6)
Saturday: Rest
Sunday: Run 40 mins (effort level 5)

WEEK SEVEN
Monday: Run 20 mins (effort level 5)
Tuesday: Rest
Wednesday: Run 5 mins (effort level
5), then repeat the following 6 times:
run 1 min (effort level 8 to 9), walk
1 min (effort level 3 to 4) (Total:
17 mins)

Thursday: Rest
Friday: Run 20 mins (effort level 7)
Saturday: Rest
Sunday: Run 45 mins (effort level 5)

WEEK EIGHT
Monday: Walk 40 mins (effort level 4)
Tuesday: Rest
Wednesday: Run 5 mins (effort level
5), then repeat the following 8 times:
run 1 min (effort level 8 to 9), walk
1 min (effort level 4) (Total: 21 mins)
Thursday: Rest
Friday: Run 30 mins (effort level
5 to 6)
Saturday: Rest
Sunday: Run 50 mins (effort level 5)

WEEK NINE
Monday: Run 25 mins (effort level 5)
Tuesday: Rest
Wednesday: Run 5 mins (effort level
5), then repeat the following 8–10
times, depending on what you can
manage: run 1 min (effort level 8 to
9), run 1 min (effort level 5) (Total:
21 to 25 mins)
Thursday: Rest
Friday: Run 20 mins (effort level 7)
Saturday: Rest
Sunday: Run 60 mins (effort level 5)

WEEK TEN
Monday: Run 30 mins (effort level 5)
Tuesday: Rest
Wednesday: Run 20 mins
(effort level 7)
Thursday: Rest
Friday: Rest
Saturday: Rest
Sunday: 10K RACE!
(effort level 5 to 6)

How to find your perfect race

When you enter your first race, it's vital to choose the right one so you have the most fun possible and don't unwittingly stumble on a speedy event that leaves you floundering. Here's how to pick the race that's right for you...

★ **Choose your distance (from 5K to 10K to half-marathon to full marathon),** then do an initial search on the internet, or buy a copy of *Runner's World* magazine and check out the race directory at the back or view it online at its fab website, www.runnersworld.co.uk.

★ **Once you've short-listed a few races, the most important things to find out are how fast and how big the race is.** You're probably better off with a slower, bigger race the first time as in small, fast races you may find yourself bringing up the rear and running on your own. It's also good to know what the ratio of male to female runners will be (if you're a woman, it's better to enter a female-friendly race rather than going it alone with a bunch of super-competitive male club runners). You can ask the race organiser these kinds of questions or, ideally, ask someone who has already run the race.

★ **Try to enter an event where there's lots of crowd support to encourage you when the going gets tough.** Some races are mobbed by spectators who'll stay for hours and cheer the very last runners over the finish line, others can be a bit of a lonely wasteland. We think you'll prefer the former!

★ **You also want to think about the practicalities.** Is the race easy to travel to? Will you have to stay somewhere overnight? How much will the whole thing – from race entry to transport – cost?

★ **Finally, think about the goodies!** Do you get a lovely shiny medal on a pink ribbon? Are you handed a goodie bag stuffed with food and drink as you cross the finish line? Will you be given a been-there-run-that souvenir T-shirt that you can proudly wear afterwards? Or do you have to make do with a pat on the back and a long walk home? After you've just run for more than half an hour, believe us, it matters!

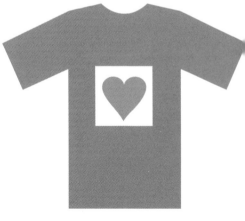

RACE DAY CHECKLIST

✔ race number
  (forget it, and forget running the race!)
✔ safety pins
✔ trainers (and a spare pair)
✔ running top/vest
✔ running jacket
✔ running shorts/bottoms
✔ sports bra
✔ knickers/underpants
✔ socks
✔ hat
✔ gloves
✔ sports watch
✔ bin bag (to keep you warm)
✔ fancy-dress outfit!
✔ change of clothes plus flip flops (great for
  tired feet)
✔ kit bag
✔ sports drink/water bottle
✔ snacks/sweets
✔ sunscreen
✔ sunglasses
✔ bumbag/mini rucksack
✔ loo roll
✔ Vaseline
✔ blister plasters
✔ painkillers
✔ cash
✔ phone
✔ camera

Mix it up

We thought we'd take a short break before launching into the half-marathon and marathon training plans, to tell you about the benefits of cross-training...

Cross-training might sound a bit technical, but it's not – it's basically just a term that means including a mix of different activities in your regular fitness programme – from cycling to swimming to weight-training. Together, these combine to bring you big fitness benefits, and even better, help improve your running. When you're a new runner and keen to improve as much as you can, as fast as you can, it's easy to think that the more you run, the better you'll get. Yet, while that's true to a certain extent, it also pays not to overdo the pavement-pounding, as it can lead to you getting injured or bored.

Which is where cross-training comes in – by adding a few different fitness activities into the mix along with your running, you can give your body a break, while working on different aspects of your fitness and strength that will complement and enhance your running. And give you great arms, a toned tummy and pert bottom in the process!

To help get you started, we asked fitness expert Jon Roberts, from Matt Roberts Personal Training (www.personaltrainer.uk.com) to give us a run-down of some of the most runner-friendly cross-training activities and some tips and advice on how to make the most of each of them. You'll never fit them all into your week, so just choose the types of cross-training that appeal the most to you and give them a go.

Swimming

Swimming is a great way to work your upper and lower body at the same time, and because you can do a variety of different strokes, you can choose to target different sets of muscles.

How will it help my running?

It'll work your heart and lungs, building up your stamina. Working against the resistance provided by the water is also a good way to strengthen your muscles. But, as a runner, one of the best things about swimming is that it allows you to reap these fitness benefits while giving your legs a welcome break from the impact they get during running.

Which strokes are best?

The best stroke for runners looking to build stronger muscles is front crawl, because of its powerful kicking action. To get results, you'll need to put some effort in – we've put together a good session for you to try (see Try this... opposite).

How often do I need to do it?

A once-a-week swim alongside regular running sessions should be enough for you to feel the benefits. If you've been injured, try swimming twice a week to maintain your fitness without overdoing it, and get you ready to start running again.

You'll also find that having a lovely relaxing swim the day after a race is a blissful way to shake off your aches and stay active without overstretching yourself.

Try this...

The best way to get the most from swimming is to work in short intervals. Try the workout below:

- Two lengths of regular front crawl, swimming at a medium/fast pace
- Two lengths of front crawl kick, using your legs only, holding a float, swimming at a fast pace
- Two lengths of front crawl using arms only, holding a float between your legs, swimming at a medium pace, with powerful strokes
- Rest for 45 seconds, then repeat

Any top tips?

- To improve your swimming, always swim with goggles. Lots of people swim with their heads out of the water, which is bad news for your neck and upper back.
- Most pools have a clock with a hand that measures seconds. Try timing yourself swimming one length and then work on beating your best time on each visit.
- You could also count how many strokes you take on a typical length, and try gradually to

decrease that number by getting more power into each stroke.

Cycling

Cycling is a fantastic aerobic activity that'll really get your heart and lungs working hard, and again will strengthen your legs without you having to do more pavement-pounding.

How will it help my running?

Cycling regularly will help you build thighs and calves of steel. It'll also build your stamina and get your heart and lungs super-fit. This is because you can cycle at a good pace on a bike without your legs getting tired too quickly, which allows you to keep your heart pumping harder and for longer periods than if you tried to sprint during a run.

What type of cycling is best?

Hill-training is a great way for runners to really strengthen their legs. Your best tactic is to find a good hill that you can tackle a few times. Try cycling up it for 5 minutes, down it for 2 minutes, and then doing it again.

If you find you get bored cycling alone, try a spinning class on static bikes at the gym. They're amazing calorie burners, and will really push your fitness to another level — just don't do one the day before a race, as you'll tire your legs out.

How often do I need to do it?

A few times a week will bring you big fitness benefits. If you struggle to fit this in, think creatively, and consider cycling to work or to the gym, or getting together with friends to make weekend cycle rides more fun.

Any top tips?

★ Visit your local bike shop and ask them to check that your bike is set up properly. Lots of people ride with their saddle too low; this can feel uncomfortable and you won't get the best body benefits from your rides.

★ Don't make the classic mistake of cycling along slowly in a really tough gear — you'll exhaust your legs without giving your heart a good workout. Instead, cycle along faster in a lower gear that allows your legs to spin more freely.

★ If you want to cycle longer distances regularly, consider getting a gel cover for your saddle and some padded shorts – they'll make you feel lots more comfy.

★ Invest in a water bottle that fits on to your bike, as it's easy to get dehydrated if you go out cycling for longer periods.

Weight-training

Weight-training is an ultra-effective way to strengthen your muscles from top-to-toe. It'll also give you the brilliant body confidence that comes when you feel strong and toned.

How will it help my running?

By building strong, toned muscles you'll get faster and reduce your risk of injury. Weight-training is also great if you're trying to lose weight — the more muscle you gain, the more calories you'll burn. As the excess weight comes off, you'll find that each and every run starts to feel easier and more enjoyable.

What type of weights are best?

Free weights (such as hand-weights or dumbbells) will encourage you to use your whole body, and will get you working harder than using fixed weights machines at the gym. If you're a total beginner, you ideally need to start with a general weight-training programme for four to six weeks, which works all the major muscle groups of the body to get you ready for lifting heavier weights. Ask a trainer to put together a programme for you, or try a weights class at a gym. If that goes well, you can then move up to lifting heavier weights (see below).

How often do I need to do it?

Once you're lifting heavier weights, you'll need to do two sessions a week to get results. Again, ask a trainer to put together a programme of key moves for you. Aim to do six to eight repetitions (reps) of each move, and to repeat each set of repetitions six to eight times, with a 2-minute rest between sets. The idea is to lift weights that are heavy enough that by the last of the reps in each set, you feel you can't do any more.

Any top tips?

★ This is one area where it's really, really worth going to a class, or having a personal training session, to learn how to do the exercises correctly. Get your technique right as soon as you start so you don't develop bad habits and injure yourself later on.

★ Don't be afraid of weights. Lots of women shy away from them because they are scared of 'bulking up', but really, you won't!

What you will gain is better posture, body confidence and body shape.

⭐ To develop strong legs, do squats and lunges holding dumbbells by your sides, or a barbell across your shoulders.

Yoga and Pilates

Going to a regular yoga or Pilates class makes you stronger and more flexible, and teaches you great body awareness. Over time you'll learn to think of your body as one whole entity that works together, rather than a series of non-connected body parts.

How will they help my running?

Both yoga and Pilates will boost your strength and work on your flexibility. Pilates has a particular focus on strengthening your abdominal muscles and back, which will help you maintain good posture when you run, and may also help make you less injury prone. Both will teach you to stretch safely, again helping to reduce the risk of injury.

Which types of yoga and Pilates are best?

All kinds will bring you benefits, so choose the type that you like best. Some yoga teachers focus a lot on breathing, others teach dynamic forms of yoga such as Ashtanga, and others take Bikram classes which are performed in heated rooms to really make you sweat and help you improve your flexibility. When it comes to Pilates, you can do mat-based Pilates, or use special equipment to work out on. See what's available in your area, and if

you don't like one class, or your instructor's teaching style, don't be afraid to swap until you find something you're more comfortable with.

How often do I need to do them?

Aim to go to a class each week, and once you're familiar with some of the moves, you can use those you find most helpful on a daily basis, perhaps before or after runs to help prepare or relax you.

Any top tips?

⭐ Leave your competitive instincts at home – these classes aren't about trying to get into a more advanced position than your neighbour; they're about focusing on how your body feels, and calming your mind.

⭐ Don't push yourself too hard too soon. You might not feel as if you're doing much in your first session, but it's deceptive, and you'll really feel it the next day.

⭐ Use the body awareness you gain in classes to really tune into how your body feels – and where you might be storing stress – while you're out on a run.

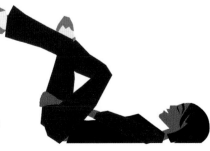

YOUR HALF-MARATHON PLAN

Who's it good for?

Aspiring marathon runners who want to gauge how far they can go. **How does it feel?** Pretty special. Complete a half-marathon and you've already done more than most people ever will.

How long will it take? Under 1:45 and you're a speed demon, about 2:00 is respectable, heading for 2:30 and you're towards the back (but that's where the interesting people hang!)

What's the plan? It's a 12-weeker designed by BUPA sports scientist Andy Ellis. If you're worried about tackling this distance, take a peek at our walk/run advice on page 162.

WEEK ONE
Monday: Rest
Tuesday: Run 30 mins (effort level 5)
Wednesday: Run 30 mins (effort level 5)
Thursday: Rest
Friday: Run 30 mins (effort level 5)
Saturday: Rest
Sunday: Run 35 mins (effort level 6). – about 5km (3 miles)!

WEEK TWO
Monday: Rest
Tuesday: Run 30 mins (effort level 5)
Wednesday: Run 30 mins (effort level 6 to 7), or test yourself with a 30-min tempo session (see overleaf)
Thursday: Rest
Friday: Run 30 mins (effort level 5)
Saturday: Rest

Sunday: Run 45 mins (effort level 6)

WEEK THREE
Monday: Rest
Tuesday: Run 30 mins (effort level 5)
Wednesday: Run 40 mins (effort level 6 to 7), or try a 40-min tempo session (see overleaf)
Thursday: Rest
Friday: Run 30 mins (effort level 5)
Saturday: Rest
Sunday: Run 55 mins (effort level 6) – about 8km (5 miles)!

WEEK FOUR
Monday: Rest
Tuesday: Run 40 mins (effort level 5)
Wednesday: Run 50 mins (effort level 6 to 7), or do a 50-min tempo session (see overleaf)
Thursday: Rest
Friday: Run 30 mins (effort level 5), or if you're feeling lively, try 28 mins of intervals (see overleaf)
Saturday: Rest
Sunday: Run 65 mins (effort level 6)

WEEK FIVE
Monday: Rest
Tuesday: Run 40 mins (effort level 5)
Wednesday: Run 30 mins (effort level 6 to 7), or do a 30-min tempo session (see overleaf)
Thursday: Rest
Friday: Run 40 mins (effort level 5), or try 28 mins of intervals (see overleaf)
Saturday: Rest
Sunday: Run 80 mins (effort level 6)

WEEK SIX
Monday: Rest
Tuesday: Run 40 mins (effort level 5)
Wednesday: Run 50 mins (effort level 6 to 7), or do a 50-min tempo session (see overleaf)
Thursday: Rest
Friday: Run 30 mins (effort level 5), or do 34 mins of intervals (see overleaf)
Saturday: Rest
Sunday: Run 90 mins (effort level 6) – about 13km (8 miles)!

WEEK SEVEN
Monday: Rest
Tuesday: Run 40 mins (effort level 5)
Wednesday: Run 40 mins (effort level 6 to 7), or do a 40-min tempo session (see overleaf)
Thursday: Rest
Friday: Run 40 mins (effort level 5) or do 34 mins of intervals (see overleaf)
Saturday: Rest
Sunday: Run 65 mins (effort level 6)

WEEK EIGHT
Monday: Rest
Tuesday: Run 40 mins (effort level 5)
Wednesday: Run 40 mins (effort level 6 to 7), or do a 40-min tempo session (see overleaf)
Thursday: Rest
Friday: Run 40 mins (effort level 5) or do 25 mins of intervals (see overleaf)
Saturday: Rest
Sunday: Run 110 mins (effort level 6) – about 16km (10 miles)!

WEEK NINE
Monday: Rest
Tuesday: Run 40 mins (effort level 5)
Wednesday: Run 50 mins (effort level 6 to 7), or do a 50-min tempo session

Thursday: Rest
Friday: Run 50 mins (effort level 5), or do 25 mins of intervals (see overleaf)
Saturday: Rest
Sunday: Run 55 mins (effort level 6)

WEEK TEN
Monday: Rest
Tuesday: Run 40 mins (effort level 5)
Wednesday: Run 40 mins (effort level 6 to 7), or do a 40-min tempo session (see overleaf)
Thursday: Rest
Friday: Run 40 mins (effort level 5), or do 25 mins of intervals (see overleaf)
Saturday: Rest
Sunday: Run 120 mins (effort level 6) – about 16km to 19km (10–12 miles)!

WEEK ELEVEN
Monday: Rest
Tuesday: Run 40 mins (effort level 5)
Wednesday: Run 40 mins (effort level 6 to 7), or do a 40-min tempo session (see overleaf)
Thursday: Rest
Friday: Run 40 mins (effort level 5), or do any of the interval sessions (overleaf)
Saturday: Rest
Sunday: Run 65 mins (effort level 6)

WEEK TWELVE
Monday: Rest
Tuesday: Run 30 mins (effort level 5)
Wednesday: Run 40 mins (effort level 6 to 7), or do a 40-min tempo session (see overleaf), optional
Thursday: Rest
Friday: Run 30 mins (effort level 5)
Saturday: Rest
Sunday: HALF-MARATHON! (effort level 5 to 6)

Tempo sessions

The 30-minute session

Warm up with 5 minutes of gentle running, then repeat the following twice: run at effort level 8 for 5 minutes, then run at effort level 5 for 5 minutes. Cool down with 5 minutes of easy running.

The 40-minute session

Warm up with 5 minutes of gentle running, then repeat the following three times: run at effort level 8 for 5 minutes, then run at effort level 5 for 5 minutes. Cool down with 5 minutes of easy running.

The 50-minute session

Warm up with 5 minutes of gentle running, then repeat the following twice: run at effort level 8 for 10 minutes, then run at effort level 5 for 10 minutes. Cool down with 5 minutes of easy running.

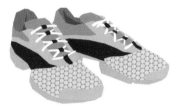

THE WORLD'S TOP 10 MARATHONS

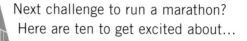

Next challenge to run a marathon?
Here are ten to get excited about...

Flora London Marathon
When: April
Its size (35,000 plus), atmosphere
and amazing crowd support make this
event oh-so special.
Visit www.london-marathon.co.uk

Boston Marathon
When: April
The world's oldest, but you have to be
fast – women aged 18–34 must be
able to run a marathon in 3:40 to
qualify. Visit www.bostonmarathon.org

Paris Marathon
When: April
A spectacular course featuring all the
major sights along the way.
Visit www.parismarathon.com

Comrades Marathon (RSA)
When: June
It's longer than a standard marathon at
89km/55.6 miles (sometimes the
distance varies), but we just had to
include this legendary South African
race! Notorious for its 12-hour cut-off
point and heroics as runners drag their
fellow comrades across the finish line.
Visit www.comrades.com

Midnight Sun Marathon (Norway)
When: June
Experience running a marathon in
broad daylight – in the middle of the
night! Visit www.msm.no/

Berlin Marathon
When: September
Flat and speedy – and beer at the
finish! Visit www.berlin-marathon.com

Marathon Du Medoc (France)
When: September
A truly unique gastro-marathon with
21 wine-tasting stops plus gourmet
food along the route.
Visit www.marathondumedoc.com

Chicago Marathon
When: October
Well organised and hassle free.
Visit www.chicagomarathon.com

New York City Marathon
When: November
A razzle-dazzle event in the Big
Apple with highly enthusiastic,
high-fiving crowds. Visit
www.ingnycmarathon.org

Reggae Marathon (Jamaica)
When: December
Run to a reggae soundtrack!
Visit www.reggaemarathon.com

YOUR MARATHON PLAN

Who's it good for?
Anyone with a slightly lunatic tendency who likes to push themselves to the limit. Exhibitionists and anyone who loves dressing up. And lots of perfectly normal people, too!
How does it feel? Sort of like arrghhh followed by hurrahhhh!!
How long will it take? Under 4 hours and you've reached the marathon holy grail, finish in 4 to 5 hours and you're about the middle of the pack. From 5 to 6 hours and beyond, you'll be having a ball in the thick of the fun runners.
What's the plan? It's adapted from an original version by running guru Professor Tim Noakes, Discovery health professor of exercise and sports science at the University of Cape Town, South Africa. Don't embark on this plan, though, until you've first worked your way through the other three given in this book.

WEEK ONE
Monday: Rest
Tuesday: Run 20 mins
Wednesday: Rest
Thursday: Run 20 mins
Friday: Run 45 mins
Saturday: Rest
Sunday: Run 20 mins

WEEK TWO
Monday: Run 40 mins
Tuesday: Run 20 mins
Wednesday: Rest
Thursday: Run 20 mins
Friday: Run 50 mins
Saturday: Rest
Sunday: Run 30 mins

WEEK THREE
Monday: Run 45 mins
Tuesday: Run 30 mins
Wednesday: Rest
Thursday: Run 30 mins
Friday: Run 50 mins
Saturday: Run 45 mins
Sunday: Rest

WEEK FOUR
Monday: Run 30 mins
Tuesday: Run 45 mins
Wednesday: Run 30 mins, or do a 30-min tempo or interval session (see overleaf)
Thursday: Run 50 mins
Friday: Rest
Saturday: Run 60 mins
Sunday: Rest

WEEK FIVE
Monday: Run 30 mins
Tuesday: Run 55 mins
Wednesday: Run 30 mins, or do a 30-min tempo or interval session (see overleaf)
Thursday: Run 55 mins
Friday: Rest
Saturday: Run 80 mins
Sunday: Rest

WEEK SIX
Monday: Run 35 mins

Tuesday: Run 60 mins
Wednesday: Run 35 mins, or do a
35-min tempo or interval session
(see overleaf)
Thursday: Run 60 mins, or rest
Friday: Run 35 mins
Saturday: Run 90 mins
Sunday: Rest

WEEK SEVEN
Monday: Run 35 mins
Tuesday: Run 70 mins
Wednesday: Run 35 mins, or do a
35-min tempo or interval session
(see overleaf)
Thursday: Run 70 mins, or rest
Friday: Run 35 mins
Saturday: Run 100 mins
Sunday: Rest

WEEK EIGHT
Monday: Run 40 mins
Tuesday: Run 80 mins
Wednesday: Run 40 mins, or do a
40-min tempo or interval session
(see overleaf)
Thursday: Run 40 mins, or rest
Friday: Run 35 mins
Saturday: Run 110 mins
Sunday: Rest

WEEK NINE
Monday: Run 40 mins
Tuesday: Run 90 mins
Wednesday: Run 40 mins, or do a
40-min tempo or interval session
(see overleaf)
Thursday: Run 90 mins, or rest
Friday: Run 40 mins
Saturday: Run 120 mins
Sunday: Rest

WEEK TEN
Monday: Run 40 mins
Tuesday: Run 90 mins
Wednesday: Run 40 mins, or do a
40-min tempo or interval session
(see overleaf)
Thursday: Run 90 mins, or rest
Friday: Run 40 mins
Saturday: Run 150 mins
Sunday: Rest

WEEK ELEVEN
Monday: Run 40 mins
Tuesday: Run 90 mins
Wednesday: Run 40 mins, or do a
40-min tempo or interval session
(see overleaf)
Thursday: Run 90 mins, or rest
Friday: Run 40 mins
Saturday: Run 100 mins
Sunday: Rest

WEEK TWELVE
Monday: Run 40 mins
Tuesday: Run 90 mins
Wednesday: Run 40 mins, or do a
40-min tempo or interval session
(see overleaf)
Thursday: Run 30 mins, or rest
Friday: Run 40 mins
Saturday: Run 80 mins
Sunday: Run 20 mins

WEEK THIRTEEN
Monday: Run 40 mins
Tuesday: Run 20 mins
Wednesday: Run 30 mins
Thursday: Rest
Friday: Rest
Saturday: Rest
Sunday: MARATHON! You did it!

Tempo sessions

The 30-minute session

Warm up with 5 minutes of gentle running, then repeat the following twice: run at effort level 8 for 5 minutes, run at effort level 5 for 5 minutes. Cool down with 5 minutes of easy running.

The 35-minute session

Warm up with 6 minutes of gentle running, then repeat the following twice: run at effort level 8 for 6 minutes, run at effort level 5 for 6 minutes. Cool down with 5 minutes of easy running.

The 40-minute session

Warm up with 5 minutes of gentle running, then repeat the following three times: run at effort level 8 for 5 minutes, run at effort level 5 for 5 minutes. Cool down with 5 minutes of easy running.

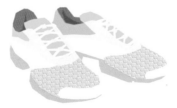

How to prepare for the big day

The week before

▐▐▐▶ Read your race pack so you know what to expect.

▐▐▐▶ Work out your journey time, then double it – things often go wrong, so leave plenty of time.

▐▐▐▶ Double-check your race number and kit. Avoid the temptation to buy and wear spanking new trainers – run in your old favourites or you risk severe blisters.

▐▐▐▶ Write or get your name printed on your T-shirt so the crowd can cheer you on.

▐▐▐▶ Plan a mile marker or landmark for your friends and family to stand at on race day, and get them to hold a sign or balloons for maximum visibility.

▐▐▐▶ Eat pasta and drink plenty of water, cut down on alcohol, get enough sleep and go easy on the running.

The night before

▐▐▐▶ Pack your bag and lay out your clothes. Use the checklist on page 149 so you don't forget anything.

▐▐▐▶ Kill your nerves with a glass of wine or beer, but no more! Drink plenty of water and stick to foods that won't upset your stomach.

▐▐▐▶ Get a good night's sleep and don't panic – you're going to be brilliant.

The big day

▐▐▐▶ Remember to enjoy yourself – it's the most important tip of all!

▐▐▐▶ If it's an early race, set your alarm so you have time to eat (and digest) breakfast. Scrambled eggs on toast a couple of hours before the starting gun makes an excellent pre-race breakfast.

▐▐▐▶ Remember to drink water en route to the race to make sure you're well hydrated.

▐▐▐▶ Have a short warm-up jog, take a quick toilet break, then stay warm and well dressed (use your old clothes or a bin bag for this) while waiting for the gun.

▐▐▐▶ Once you're off, stick to your pace and don't let the excitement of the big day make you run too fast – listen to how your body is feeling.

▐▐▐▶ Be careful at the drinks stations – watch out for people in front of you stopping or swerving sharply.

▐▐▐▶ Drink steadily and sensibly during the race. If they're giving out bottles of water, carry one with you; if the drink is in a cup, squeeze it into a funnel shape to make drinking on the move easier.

▐▐▐▶ Assess how you're feeling at the halfway point – do you need to slow down or speed up?

▐▐▐▶ If you're tired, run at the edge of the pack and closer to the crowds so you'll get more support.

▐▐▐▶ Smile broadly every time you see a race photographer so you'll look great in your official photographs.

▐▐▐▶ Save some energy so you can run towards the finish line looking and feeling fantastic.

▐▐▐▶ After you've stopped, stretch, put on some warm clothes, and refuel with drinks and food. Try to keep moving as much as possible so your muscles don't seize up. Then pat yourself on the back – and enjoy the glory!

Don't forget to walk the walk!

Remember, the walk/run technique you learnt when first starting to run can come in handy for longer distances, too...

The walk-break method is the most powerful tool that American fitness expert and author Jeff Galloway has ever found for improving marathon performance and reducing injury. Galloway, who has coached more than 100,000 marathoners using his walk/run training schedules, says, 'Most runners will record significantly faster times when they take walk breaks because they don't slow down at the end of a long run. The early walk breaks help combat fatigue, while the later ones help reduce the amount of damage your muscles suffer in a race.'

how long, how often?

Galloway recommends taking walk breaks right from the start of a race (see the ratios on the opposite page for suggestions on how long they should be) until you get to about 30km (mile 19) in the marathon. After that point, you can either shorten them or even phase them out altogether (because by then you'll be pretty certain you're going to finish!). And don't forget to practise taking walk breaks when you're training. Galloway says you can omit them in your shorter training runs if you like, but should include them on your longer runs so you can work out the ratio that's best for you, can practise timing yourself and can get used to walking fast (it's not as easy as it sounds!).

So don't ditch everything The 60-Second-Secret Plan taught you – it may get you through that marathon with less pain, more fun and perhaps even more quickly!

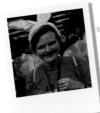

66 I'd done two marathons and tried different strategies to get me round, with varying degrees of success (and distress!). And then, in the Paris Marathon, I had a major breakthrough. I injured my knee in training and the night before the race I was convinced I wouldn't finish, but I came across a suggestion in the marathon booklet that struggling runners should take walk breaks right from the start. I tried it and was amazed at the results. Running for 15 minutes and walking for 5 broke the race into manageable sections. I spent the walk breaks snacking and chatting, and found they really rested my legs. Best of all, I bettered my previous marathon time, when I'd run all the way, by a whopping 10 minutes!
Lisa Jackson, 40, co-author of *Running Made Easy* 99

WALK/RUN RATIOS

Marathon time goal: 6 hours+	1 minute walking, then 1 minute running
Marathon time goal: 5:30 to 6 hours	1 minute walking, then 1 to 2 minutes' running
Marathon time goal: 5 hours to 5.29	1 minute walking, then 3 to 5 minutes' running
Marathon time goal: 4:30 to 4:59	1 minute walking, then 4 to 6 minutes' running
Marathon time goal: 4 hours to 4:29	1 minute walking, then 7 to 8 minutes' running
Marathon time goal: 3:51 to 3:59	55 seconds' walking every mile
Marathon time goal: 3:41 to 3:50	45 seconds' walking every mile
Marathon time goal: 3:30 to 3:40	35 seconds' walking every mile
Marathon time goal: 3:22 to 3:29	30 seconds' walking every mile
Marathon time goal: 3:16 to 3:21	20 seconds' walking every mile
Marathon time goal: 3:08 to 3:15	15 seconds' walking every mile
Marathon time goal: 2:50 to 3:07	10 seconds' walking every mile

Marathon magic

Just about everyone who has run a marathon agrees it's a day in a million. We quizzed some proud finishers about taking on the ultimate challenge...

❝Running the London Marathon with my husband was certainly an experience – we went through every emotion in those 4½ hours, from quiet tension at the start line, laughing and joking at how clever we were when we passed the halfway mark, a huge row at 30km (19 miles) over our pace (when we decided it was probably best not to talk for a few miles), to **holding hands and literally falling into each other's arms as we crossed the finish line.** It was such an amazing feeling. The crowd support is unbelievable, it's like getting a little shot of adrenaline. After weeks of really tough training when I thought about giving up nearly every day, I had one of the best and most memorable days of my life.' **Rebecca Frank, 29, deputy editor, *Zest*, London**

'I'd always trained for the New York City Marathon listening to music on my Walkman, and I found that really fast dance music helped me keep to a pace. So when I went over to America to run the marathon all on my own, I asked two friends to make me a tape of songs to listen to during the race, and asked them to speak on it and cheer me on. They chose things I'd never have thought of – like 'Reach For The Stars' by S Club 7 – which kept surprising me, and **they even said things like, "Come on, Rach, you can do it" between songs, which was just like having pats on the back all the way round**. When I finished the race, I wanted the whole of New York to lift me on their shoulders because it was such an achievement for me!' **Rachel Armitage, 29, charity worker, Sheffield**

'A route that takes you through herds of zebra and acacia groves must make the Lewa Downs Marathon in Kenya one of the most remarkable races in the world. Sunrise finds herds of elephant and rhinoceros along the roadside and prides of lions asleep on the track. The race begins early, with helicopters, spotter planes and rangers fanning out in the pre-dawn light to make sure any dangerous wildlife has moved away from the roads. **Game rangers keep a watchful eye on proceedings as the runners, walkers and strollers enjoy spectacular views of Mount Kenya** – as well as herds of game at the roadside. I cannot think of any better way to appreciate the natural beauty of the African savannah grasslands.' **Mukesh Kerai, 32, systems engineer, Sydney, Australia**

'In New York I'd got injured by 29km (18 miles) and was really suffering. Just in front of me, **I saw this guy running with an artificial leg. I slotted in behind him, and just kept telling myself, "If he can do it, I can do it."** It became my mantra. He knew exactly where I was at, and how I was feeling, and he got me round the final kilometres. It turned out he was Chris Moon, a really famous runner who lost part of his right leg and his right arm while clearing landmines in Mozambique. Meeting someone like that, who's overcome all the odds and who raises so much money every time he runs, was like bumping into an angel.'
Shelly Vella, 37, fashion director, *Cosmopolitan*, London

'I decided to run the London Marathon as a personal challenge. It was something I'd watched friends do and never dreamed I'd manage myself, but I built up by doing short races and realised I *could* do it. I was never fast — my goal was just to run the whole way, and I did — even though sometimes I was at a snail's pace! On the start line I felt terrified, but as the gun went off, all my panic melted away. Running along, I had such an amazing, sociable time, singing and chatting to people.

I had a wobble around 17 miles, but some friends who were watching ran alongside me and got me back on track, and from then on, I knew I'd make it. Running for the finish line, the tune to *Chariots of Fire* was playing in my head, and I wanted those moments to last forever. I finished in 5 hours, and floated around on a high for days. I'd astounded myself and my friends!'
Lindsay Cunningham, 34, teacher, Hampshire

'I ran the London Marathon four weeks after having an ovary removed. Standing on the start line, I couldn't believe I'd made it. **I ran with my sister Louise, and finished in just over 4½ hours with a few tears and big hugs along the way**. It was only a month after the race, when I'd come down off my high, that the impact of what I'd been through really hit me. I'm convinced that being so fit and healthy is what helped me recover so quickly from the operation, and having the marathon to focus on helped me through what could have been a really traumatic time.
Rebecca Lake, 31, PA, York 〞

" They say life begins at 40 – or at least my running career did! I live a stone's throw from the start of the London Marathon and every year I found myself completely choked up by this amazing event. **The year I hit 40, I applied for a place, despite having only ever run for about 15 minutes at a time and being known as the Queen of the Black Cab!** My first run outside was on New Year's Eve and I ached for Britain while everyone else celebrated. But things got better – I had chickenpox in my mid-30s and had tried everything to ease the post-viral fatigue that dogged me for years. Miraculously, running magicked away all the back and shoulder problems it had left me with. Thanks to my job, I even found myself swapping running tips with Alastair Campbell a few days before the London Marathon. And it really was one fantastically memorable day.'
Jackie Graveney, 41, PR executive, London

'I and a few running friends have been training disabled people to run for quite a few years. It has given us untold rewards and enjoyment to see them develop and go from despair to becoming pillars of their communities. I took my first blind runner through the 89km (55.6-mile) Comrades Marathon in South Africa in 1985, and he moaned for almost the entire 10½ hours as I pulled and tugged him up the hills. I kept him cool by pouring cups of cold water over his head every now and again. When I told him he was near the end of the race, he managed to get what he thought was a cup of water and promptly poured it over my head as a token of appreciation for what I'd been doing for him. Unfortunately, the cup he'd been handed was full of warm Coca-Cola! I was not at all happy with him, as you can imagine!'
Denis Tabakin, 62, footwear consultant, Johannesburg, South Africa

---

'If someone had told me a few years ago that I'd be lining up at the start of the 2002 London Marathon next to Paula Radcliffe, I would have laughed in their face. Since my first running experience had seen me struggling to make it twice round a field only a few years before, this scenario seemed extremely unlikely. But amazingly, even though I started running late in life, **I improved really fast and was soon good enough to line up with the elite women!** I can now run the sorts of times I initially would only have dreamed of (my marathon personal best is 3:01). I've gained so much from running – friends, a husband (I met him at the running club!), a leaner body, a much healthier attitude to life, and, of course, my five minutes of fame as I lined up in the London marathon next to Paula Radcliffe and waved to my mum!'
Pippa Major, 37, e-commerce development manager, Surrey

'What I love about doing a marathon is that the buzz and sense of achievement never go away. **The memory of turning the corner of the Mall into the final straight of the London Marathon and seeing the clock with those big yellow digits ticking over is as vivid as the memory of when my daughter was born** and laid on my chest. It sounds disproportionate, but the months of commitment involved make finishing a marathon a very special moment.'
Emma Simpson, 31, designer, London

'I'd already done a few marathons and triathlons, and so finally worked up the bottle to tackle the Ironman UK Triathlon. It starts with a 2.4 mile swim, then a 112 mile bike ride, and you finish by running a marathon. Amazingly I felt relatively OK when I got off the bike after 7½ hours of cycling, and started running – the sun was shining, and my sisters were playing the theme tune to *Rocky* on a little portable CD player as I set off!

I ran the first 13 miles in about 2 hours, which I was delighted with, but by then I was running out of energy. I knew there was a photographer on the course so I kept going until I'd passed him as I didn't want to get snapped walking! But then, I ended up walking the next 10 miles. By now we'd been on the go for over 11 hours and it was totally dark. But, finally, with 2 miles to go, I started running again. **I wanted to do it in under 15 hours, and even managed to put in a sprint at the end, finishing in 14:49**. I celebrated by swapping Lucozade for lager. Although the training took over my life for a while, I do think I'd like to do another one as I really enjoyed feeling that fit. Next time, I'd be aiming to finish in under 14 hours, though!'
James Danaher, 32, lawyer, London

'It's weird, but for some reason I can't recall any of the bad bits of the Edinburgh Marathon, only the good ones. Whereas I find it really hard to remember how battered my legs and knees felt, the memories that never seem to fade are **the haunting sound of bagpipes in the mist at the start**, seeing the magnificent Forth Rail Bridge in the distance and the exhilaration as I crossed the finish line.
Graham Williams, 44, intelligence analyst, London 99

One minute everything's going brilliantly and you're enjoying your running, and the next minute disaster strikes. Maybe you've run out of steam, hit a motivation crisis, picked up an injury, or simply stopped seeing results? Well, don't panic because we know how to pick you up and set you back on your feet...

9

get over it

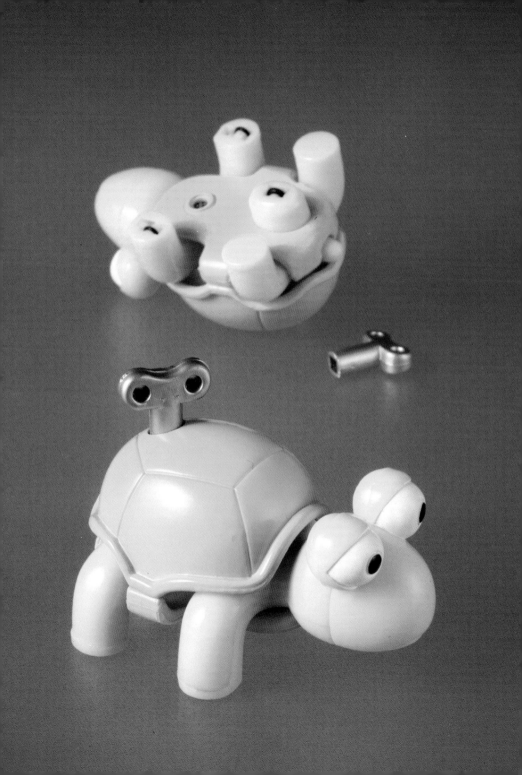

Help! Something's gone wrong!

As a new runner, it can feel very worrying to hit any kind of an obstacle. What exactly are you meant to do the first time you feel your enthusiasm for running start to fade, you pull a muscle, or you feel your fitness is stagnating rather than improving?

Well, the first thing is to realise that you're not alone – just about every runner in the world has hit the odd brick wall and had to learn how to climb over it – and you can, too. To make it that bit easier for you, we've quizzed some top experts to come up with the advice you need to help you through three common crises.

How to get over a motivation crisis

So you're having a motivation crisis? You've been running for a while, you were chuffed at your progress and then life got in the way; you skipped one run, then another, and now it's been a month since your trainers tasted tarmac. And it feels like an uphill struggle to get going again. But don't despair: you have a secret weapon – your unconscious mind – at your disposal. Learn to tap into it through some simple self-hypnosis techniques and it can get you right back on track.

There's no need to be nervous about trying self-hypnosis – what you probably don't realise is that you're just as capable as a hypnotherapist of taking yourself into the supremely relaxed, but mentally alert, state known as the trance state. During trance your unconscious mind (the place where all your memories, behaviours and attitudes are stored) is dominant and you can use visualisations and affirmations to help unblock your motivation crisis, to change your self-limiting beliefs and achieve your running goals. Here Lisa, the co-author of this book, who's also a clinical hypnotherapist, explains how to practise self-hypnosis:

1 Find a quiet place and sit or lie down comfortably. Close your eyes and start counting from ten to one, silently saying a number each time you breathe out, while noticing any tension flowing out of your body.

2 When you reach one, you'll be in a light trance state. Now imagine yourself in your favourite place of relaxation – experience it in the greatest possible detail (sounds, smells, sights) and become aware of how profoundly relaxed you feel.

3 Now you can do one of the three things explained below:

★ Start reciting a mantra to yourself. Make sure it's positive and exciting, such as 'I love the way running makes me feel' or 'I am motivated, fit and fabulous!'
★ Imagine yourself lacing up your trainers and going for the best run of your life. See how effortlessly

your body moves (and how big your smile is!). Imagine every detail of this glorious run. Then see yourself returning home, flushed with pride, and treating yourself to a reward – taste that ice-cold beer or feel the bubbles in the bubble bath tickle your skin. Imagine your sporting hero/ine during a winning performance, and then float into their body and see yourself running in exactly the same way.

4 Now it's time to wake yourself up by counting from one to ten, silently saying each number as you breathe in. When you open your eyes at ten you'll feel optimistic and refreshed – and raring to run!

5 For best results, practise self-hypnosis twice daily for between 5 and 20 minutes. Remember, self-hypnosis is a skill and you'll get better and better at it (and go into a deeper trance) each time.

How to get over a fitness plateau

In the early days of any running career, you're likely to progress in leaps and bounds. As your fitness improves, the pounds drop off, and your energy doubles, you feel fantastic, and so you should! But, after a few months, something alarming happens. You stop making great progress, and start to feel as if you're stagnating. Runs stop getting easier, and start to feel – well, a bit boring instead. Your weight stops dropping. And your motivation starts to slide.

But this isn't a reason to give up and decide that running has stopped

working for you. All that's happened is that you've hit a fitness plateau, which is something that can derail any of us if we don't shake up our running routine regularly.

'People are amazed and mystified when they first hit a plateau, because they're not expecting it', explains top personal trainer Jane Wake (www.body-a-wake.com), whose work involves coaching celebrity clients through the London Marathon, and acting as a fitness consultant to Nike.

'Think of it like learning to drive a car – at first it feels like hard work but quickly it becomes automatic and effortless. The same thing happens when you run – your body becomes more and more effective at it, the number of calories you burn goes down, and you stop seeing improvements.'

Time for a shake-up

The way to break out of a plateau is by taking your running to the next level and giving your body a new set of challenges that will increase your fitness. Trainers call this following a 'periodised' programme, which basically means that every six to eight weeks you shake up your programme and add new elements to it.

We've given you a range of programmes in this book, from a beginners' walk-to-run programme, to a 10K and ultimately a marathon plan. If you work through these, building your distances gradually and adding in the different types of sessions we recommend, you'll continue to challenge yourself and avoid the dreaded plateau.

But, just in case you don't want to follow such detailed plans and don't harbour any marathon ambitions, we also asked Jane to come up with another option. So, if you're feeling stuck in a running rut, try following the plan below for six to eight weeks, and see the difference it makes. It's based on doing three different runs each week.

1 The short, sharp run
This is your most intense run, and it'll feel like an effort level of up to 8 out of 10. Each time you go out, your aim is to run for the same amount of time – say 20 minutes – but to cover more ground so you run farther. Either run a straight route, so you can literally aim to make it to the next tree or lamp-post, or try doing interval training, and aim to race farther than before on each burst of effort.

2 The moderate run
This is a run of about 5K (3 miles), where you aim to build in lots of variety, and to hit an effort level of up to 6 out of 10. Make sure you're constantly throwing in new terrains, such as hills, and add variety, such as circuits of body-conditioning moves. So, for example, you might run for a few minutes, then do step-ups onto a park bench, run some more, then do walking lunges or a set of squats, then run up a hill, and so on.

3 The longer run
Take this run at a steady pace that you can maintain and, each week, add another 500m to it. How long your run ends up will depend on your starting point, but if, for example, you start off capable of running 8K (5 miles), you need to work up to

covering 10K (6 miles) within about four weeks. In terms of effort level, it'll probably start off feeling like a 4 out of 10, but as you come to the end of your run, it may feel more like an 8 out of 10.

How to get over an injury
It's very frustrating when an injury puts you out of action and gets in the way of your beloved running plan. And it's something that's happened to lots of us, for all different reasons – ranging from the way our bodies are built, to falls, accidents and the lifestyle challenges we face.

'Many of the injuries I see aren't caused by the actual running, but are down to the fact that we all lead such sedentary lives and then expect to go off and do very energetic bouts of exercise without warming up first and being well prepared,' explains chartered physiotherapist Sammy Margo, who runs a successful London practice (www.sammymargo.com).

The first time you tear a muscle or get pulled up short by knee pain, it can feel like a major blow, but there's no reason you can't get over it, given the right treatment and advice. What follows here are Sammy's top tips for getting you running again. If, however, you need information on diagnosing and treating a specific injury, you need to see a doctor or physiotherapist before you try following them.

'Once you're 80% recovered from an injury and you've had the okay from a physiotherapist, you're fine to start running again,' advises Sammy. Her five-step plan should help you to ease back in.

1 Wrap up warm

Keep the injured area warm and well supported when you first venture back out. If, for example, you've had a groin strain, try wearing cycling shorts under your tracksuit bottoms.

2 Check your trainers

Just after an injury is a good moment to check your trainers. If you're wearing a pair that are worn out or aren't giving you enough support, you put more stress on your knees, lower back and pelvis. These areas are more vulnerable than normal due to your injury. The general rule is to change your trainers about every 600 miles, which, if you run 12 miles a week, is roughly one new pair a year.

3 Go soft

When you're returning from an injury, avoid pavements and other hard surfaces, and head for softer surfaces such as grass to help ease the impact and strain on your body. Just be on the lookout for potholes or obstacles that could trip you. Regular walk breaks will also help you come back more comfortably.

4 Be realistic

Don't try to make up for lost time when you return to running. Instead, realise you'll have to build back up slowly. The first time you go out, simply walk for 3 minutes, run for 1 minute, walk for another 3 minutes – then turn and head for home. Yes, that's really all! The next day, if you feel okay, repeat the same pattern. On the third day walk for 4 minutes, run for 2, walk for 4 and then call it a day. You really do need to build up gradually, and never ignore any pain you may feel.

5 Make time for your tum

When you're recovering from an injury and running less than normal, use the extra time to devote to working on your core stability – namely making your lower abdominals and pelvic floor as strong as possible. The better your core stability, the less injury prone you'll be, and the more your running performance will improve. Think of your body as a crane; having good core stability is the equivalent of having a strong, fixed base to the crane, which allows the arm of the crane to move freely and with good control. If, on the other hand, the base of the crane – or the centre of your body – is wobbly and unstable, the arm of the crane – or the movements of your arms and legs – will be wobbly and uncontrolled too! Your best bet is to go to Pilates classes where you can learn specific exercises that will help to improve your core stability.

○ ○ ○ Want to hear something amazing? Then read the stories of these nine truly exceptional runners from around the world who were so determined to run that they overcame obstacles that would have stopped most ordinary people in their tracks. They're living proof that where there's a will, there's a way...

10
get amazed

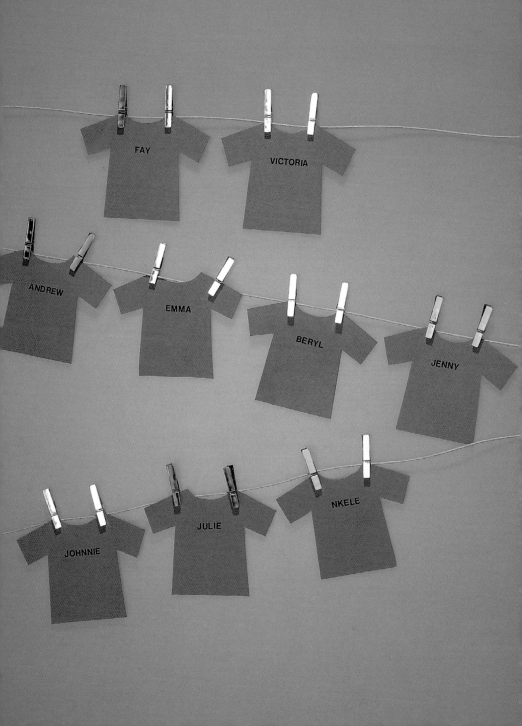

'RUNNING HELPED ME BEAT ALCOHOLISM'

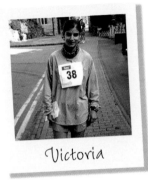

Victoria

While she was a teenager, VICTORIA BROCKHURST, 29, from London, battled addictions to alcohol and Valium, but now she faces entirely different challenges as she tackles some of the world's toughest ultra-marathons

66 I started drinking at 13. I experimented with alcohol at a party, and from the very first time I tasted it, I drank until I passed out. I wasn't very happy at that time and alcohol made me feel more relaxed and extrovert. By the time I was 16, I was drinking two litres of vodka a day and my health had deteriorated dramatically. My liver was enlarged, I had a bleeding stomach ulcer and food made me feel sick. I smelled of alcohol even when I wasn't drinking because of the vodka I was sweating out. Things got so bad that, at the age of 17, I was asked to leave school and undergo a home detox supervised by my mum. I had to take Antabuse (a medication that makes you violently ill if you drink alcohol) and was prescribed Valium to help control the shaking and horrifying hallucinations that were the side effects of going cold turkey. I succeeded in giving up drinking (though I developed an addiction to Valium) and four months later was allowed back at school to sit my exams. However, the day after my A-levels, I began drinking again.

The turning point came when, aged 19, I was admitted to A&E after I'd cut my finger while drinking. I heard

'I knew I had to find something to replace the role alcohol had played in my life and I chose running'

the doctor telling a nurse I was 'a drunk' and that's when I said to myself, 'I don't want to do this any more.' A few days later, I checked into a rehab centre where I received treatment for my addictions.

When I came out of rehab, I knew I had to find something to replace the role alcohol had played in my life. I'd always been sporty, so I chose running. I didn't really enjoy my first session as my body was still very weak after everything it had been through in the detox. But I don't do things by halves, so I took to running in the way I had to drinking – I ran a lot! I decided to start racing, and over the next five years I went from doing 5Ks to completing the London Marathon.

I'd go for long runs, six days a week. As an alcoholic, you're warned

'Everything always seems better after a run. You could say that running has taught me to be happy'

that when you stop drinking you might try to replace alcohol with something else. I knew I had the ability to go overboard with my running and so had to be careful not get too obsessed.

new life

I worked as a chef after leaving school but after getting so into running, I retrained as a personal trainer and now run a fitness company. I fundraise for Sport Against Addiction, which works with the charity Action On Addiction, to raise awareness of addiction, and I hope my story will help others beat their addictions, too.

A few years ago, I competed in the Marathon des Sables, a 243K (151-mile) race that takes place over six days in the Moroccan desert and is often billed as 'the world's toughest foot race'. An unexpected bonus was that it led to me meeting my future husband Dan while doing an 87K (54-mile) race in preparation for it. He held a gate open for me along the route and when I saw him at the finish, we agreed to pair up for a few more training sessions. Six weeks later, we did the Marathon des Sables together in scorching temperatures that often reached 40°C. We were elated to

finish, particularly as my dad was waiting at the finish line – and five months later Dan and I got engaged!

'The Marathon of Britain was our next challenge. It involved running 282K (175 miles) over six days. The weather was really hot, and the hilly course meant it felt even tougher than the Marathon des Sables. Then came the Trans 333 in Egypt, a 360K (224-mile) race when I ran virtually non-stop for about three days. I was too afraid to sleep because every time I lay down and shut my eyes, I was worried that I wouldn't be able to start running again! It was scary, but exhilarating, being on my own in the desert.

I'm just so thankful for what running's done for me. It's helped me stay sober for ten years by giving me new goals to aim for, and has also given me belief in myself. I used to drink when I was sad or depressed, but now I go running. Everything always seems better after a run. In fact, you could say that running has taught me to be happy! **99**

How Victoria did it

Motivation tip: 'Join a club or run with a running partner – it'll help you push yourself harder and having an appointment means you're less likely not to go.'
Training tip: 'It's OK to walk! Don't give yourself a hard time about it if you have to – just remind yourself that it's better to walk than to stop!'

'I LOST OVER HALF MY BODYWEIGHT'

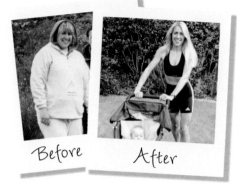

Before   After

**Weighing 121kg (19st 1lb),
JULIE PRINCE, 37, from Reading
couldn't even climb the stairs
without getting out of breath.
Now she's an incredible 62kg
(9st 11lb) lighter – all thanks
to running**

" At my biggest, I was a size 24 and weighed 121kg (19st 1lb). I got dizzy just walking up stairs, and thought I'd never, ever be able to run. Just 18 months later, having taken up running and changed my eating habits, I'd lost 62kg (9st 11lb) and slimmed down to a size 10! The change in my body and my health is unbelievable – I'm half my previous size and I've found I'm actually good at something I never thought I could do in a million years.

I was first put on a diet aged ten by my GP, and by secondary school I was a size 16 and one of the biggest girls in my class. I slimmed down to 76kg (12st) for my wedding day but soon piled the weight back on again. Things got worse when my husband's job moved us to Aberdeen in Scotland. Feeling isolated, lonely and bored, I took refuge in comfort eating.

I found a new job as a teacher but the pupils ridiculed me about my size and one nicknamed me 'Titanic'. I was still reasonably confident as my husband never criticised my weight and complimented me on other things like my hair and nails. However, my size really hit home when I couldn't do up a size 22 blazer I'd bought for an interview and could barely get a bath towel to meet round my body. I

'I got dizzy just walking up a flight of stairs... and could barely get a bath towel to meet round my body'

remember crying because I couldn't find anything to wear to a party, and my husband making me a dress himself to try to help me feel better.

I finally started losing weight in an attempt to shape up for a friend's wedding, having got the shock of my life after standing on the scales and watching them tip to 121kg (19st 1lb). I'm quite tall – 1.73m (5ft 8in) – but I realised half of me had to go! I didn't begin running straightaway – instead, I started very gently with swimming and walking, and just eating healthy meals rather than following a diet. It took me nine months to lose the first 32kg (5st), and it was at this stage that I discovered running.

My husband's job had taken us to Tunisia, and we were living in a village

and I went from losing 0.25kg (½lb) a week to losing just over 1kg (2½lb) a week. It was an amazing motivator to have found something that had such an effect on my body.

Although at the start losing 19kg (3st) didn't feel as if it made a huge difference because I had so very far to go, by now I was noticing significant changes.

'The first few runs were really hard – I was at the back and hated feeling so breathless and under pressure'

in a compound with security guards and a 750m (½-mile) track that ran right round it. One of our friends bet me that I couldn't even make it round the track once. I set off on my own to prove him wrong, and ran six laps, very slowly, stopping between each one. Inspired, my husband and I decided to join the group of Brits in our village who were training to do their first half-marathon.

tricks and tactics

The first few runs were really hard. Although I wasn't the biggest in the group, I was at the back, and I hated feeling so breathless and under pressure to keep up. We combined jogging and walking, going round and round the track, often late at night because of the heat. To help me stay motivated, I used a workbook that I'd take everywhere with me. I wrote down every run I did, everything I ate, every compliment anyone paid me, and the date when I got out of the seriously overweight bracket of the weight chart. I even drew a weight-loss graph to keep me on track. Once I started running, the line on the graph began to plummet,

My stomach was slimming down and I remember how overjoyed I felt when I fitted into a pair of size 20 white jeans – I thought I was the cat's whiskers, even though I needed my husband's help to squeeze me into them!

I ran my first race about five months later when I came back to England for a summer holiday, and it felt like a big milestone. I was very, very nervous and unwittingly had chosen a really fast 10K (6-mile) race that was full of good club runners. I'd made my way to the very front as I thought I'd need a bit of a head start, and ended up getting elbowed by all

'I began to slim down and when I fitted into a pair of size 20 jeans thought I was the cat's whiskers'

the fast runners trying to get by! Running towards the finish line, I heard one of the marshals say I was last, so I put on a spurt and beat the two other ladies in front of me to come in third from last. Although I'd not exactly picked an ideal first race to try, I was on a real high about my time – a very respectable 56 minutes – and felt very proud of myself.

179

Next came the half-marathon I'd trained for with the group. It took place in Florence, Italy. I'd reached my goal weight (63.6kg/10st) and was feeling brilliant. I already knew I was going to make the distance as I'd run 30 laps of our track in the compound – the equivalent of a half-marathon. But I was desperate to get round in under 2 hours, which I did, and achieving that goal set me off wanting to try to run the Flora London Marathon in under 4 hours.

Something else that made the half-marathon feel very special was that just afterwards we found out I was expecting our daughter Helena. I'd run the race while pregnant without even realising it! I kept on running gently throughout my pregnancy and afterwards I lost 6.4kg (1st) more than my pre-pregnancy weight, partly because I was breastfeeding, and partly because Iwas training for the marathon.

perfect day
By now, we'd moved back to England, and I would set off with Helena in her running buggy, run the 6.5K (4 miles) into town, have my treat, which was a café latte, then run home again. I loved the variety of being able to run to visit other places rather than having just to run round in circles in the compound. I also used the running as thinking and planning time.

I stuck to my training religiously for the marathon, and consequently everything went right for me on the day and I finished in 3 hours and 51 minutes. It was truly brilliant, and even now, thinking about the day and the atmosphere sends tingles down my spine.

Running has been great in other ways, too. I'm confident enough to go running in shorts and a crop top, and I can buy size 10 clothes off the rail and wear whatever I want because my weight has now stabilised at 59kg (9st 4lb). It's also done so much for my health and I have lots more energy.

slow but sure
Now I'm keen to run another marathon soon, but recently I've also been helping some of my friends to start running, explaining to them how important it is to start off slowly. When they claim they can't even run to the end of the road, I tell them that's how I felt as well. I firmly believe that being patient is the key to both learning to run and losing weight. Lots of people want a fast solution, and the more weight they have to lose, the quicker they want to lose it. But if you learn to go slow, you can achieve anything you want to – I'm living proof!

How Julie did it
Motivation tip: 'Keep a record of the progress you make – I wrote absolutely everything down. I even devised a sticker system, awarding myself a gold star every time I completed an exercise session.'
Diet tip: 'I try to copy the way my husband eats, to keep me relaxed about food and stop me falling back into the "I'm a big person trying to lose weight" mentality. If he wants a biscuit, he goes ahead and has one, and so do I.'

'RUNNING HAS BEEN MY SAVIOUR'

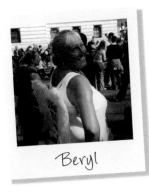

Beryl

Having suffered years of severe depression, BERYL THOMAS, 52, became a virtual prisoner in her own home. Now a keen runner, she's fully recovered, 28.6kg (4st 7lb) lighter and pounding the streets of Darwen, England, wearing angel wings and an ear-to-ear grin

❝ I'd always been a really bouncy, happy-go-lucky person, but about ten years ago I became severely depressed. It was partly due to money worries, and I'd also taken on too much in my job as a childminder. I had to give up work, and I'd sit at home rocking and staring into space, unable to stop crying. I tried everything from Prozac to electric shock therapy, but nothing seemed to work, and eventually things became so bad that I even tried to take an overdose. I became incredibly withdrawn, and if someone knocked on my front door, I'd get down on my hands and knees and hide behind the sofa rather than answer it.

It was a terrible time, not just for me, but also for my husband, Howard, my twin daughters, Katie and Kelly, now 22, and my son, Anthony, now 17, who had to go through the trauma of seeing me so ill. It got so bad that I couldn't leave the house, and the only time I'd go out was to go food shopping with Howard. I was like a

'I'd get down on my hands and knees and hide behind the sofa rather than answer a knock at my front door'

frightened child, clinging to his arm and having panic attacks.

After almost ten years of battling against depression, things finally changed for me in May 2001. It was getting light very early in the morning and, although I can't quite explain why, I suddenly felt I wanted to get out of the house. I got up at 5.30am and went for a walk on the edge of the moors where I knew no one would be about, never giving my safety a second thought. Although going out alone felt very frightening, the sense of freedom I experienced being away from those four walls was amazing. I realised from day one that getting outside and getting moving gave me a high.

After I'd been out a few times, I started to think I could try to run a few steps. At first, I could manage only ten steps before my chest felt as if it was going to explode. My medication and comfort eating had made my weight soar to 95.5kg (15st) and I was wearing a dress size 22, so I found running terribly hard and got very red in the face. But I saw it as a challenge and began counting how many steps I could manage, aiming to run for 100 steps. The first time that I could run all the way back to my house, I was literally jumping for joy.

I also started going to meetings at Weight Watchers, taking my daughter

'The first time that I could run all the way back to my house, I was literally jumping for joy '

Kelly along for moral support, but I was very nervous and sat right at the back of the class not wanting to be noticed or say anything. It was a slow process, but the running helped my confidence grow day by day, and by July, I'd plucked up the courage to enter a race – the Great Women's Run in Manchester. It's a wonderful race that gives you the chance to run down Coronation Street where the soap opera is filmed. Although it was only 8K (5 miles), it took me well over two hours to finish.

After a while, the combination of dieting and exercising began to work and I got slimmer all over. I started losing a couple of pounds each week and found that even my neck and feet changed shape! The more weight I lost, the more confident, happy and in control I felt, and I even managed to go back to work.

One day close to Christmas, I was in town shopping and I saw some angel wings in a shop. I don't know what hit me, but I just thought I'd stick them on my back when I was out running for a bit of a laugh. My son Anthony was horrified and said I wasn't to go out in them, and to be honest I felt pretty silly the first time I wore them. My heart was really pounding as I put them on, and I even wore sunglasses and a cap so no one would be able to recognise me!

The reaction I got was amazing, as by this time I was running all over town and on busy roads. Drivers would toot their horns at me and workmen couldn't believe their eyes. My daughter Kelly made little signs for me on the computer to wear on my back – one said 'Angel In Training' and another said 'Looking For Heaven'. The more I ran, the more daring I became. I collected a whole selection of wings – ones with

'I saw some angel wings in a shop and thought it would be a bit of a laugh to wear them when running'

feathers, diamanté and lace. Even the local radio station spotted me and ran a competition to find out who I was. When it tracked me down, they interviewed me on air about what I was up to. I was amazed at the way the whole thing had snowballed, and just had to explain I was wearing them for fun. Even so, I earned the nickname 'The Angel of the North', after the huge statue of an angel that stands on a hillside outside Newcastle upon Tyne.

In 2002 I ran the Great Women's Run in Manchester again, this time with my wings on. My daughter Katie was even inspired to run the race with me, though she'd never run before. By this time, I'd lost about 28.6kg (4st 7lb) and was feeling great. I got a place right at the front with all the elite runners and set off with them with a really serious look on my face (wearing my wings!) because I wanted to do a really good time.

guardian angel

Soon after the race, I finally came off my medication and decided I wanted to do the Flora London Marathon the following year. I was determined to do it as a celebration of my twin daughters' 21st birthday, and to raise money for the neonatal department that had looked after them when they'd been born prematurely. The day I found out I'd got a place in the marathon through the ballot, I was literally whooping for joy. I did all of my training with my angel wings on – by then, they had just become a part of me. They were really appropriate, too, as I'd become convinced that I had a guardian angel watching over me, keeping me safe and motivated.

learning to fly

On marathon day all my nerves had gone and I was on a complete high, wearing my wings with feathers on and a sign saying 'Learning To Fly'. Although I found it hard and got very tired and dehydrated, somehow I found the will to keep going. The crowds were brilliant. I hadn't known

you were meant to write your name on your T-shirt so people could shout for you, but it didn't matter – they all just shouted, 'Go on Angel!' All I could do was cry, and not quietly – I was really wailing! When I saw the finish line, it was like Christmas and birthdays all rolled into one. I crossed the line beaming for all the photographs!

leading the way

Running really has been my saviour. Looking back, I can't believe how poorly I'd been and how much running turned things round for me. My husband teases me that I've now got a bony bottom, and I can even fit into my daughters' clothes! I've turned into a kind of running Pied Piper – other women ask if they can run with me and turn to me for advice. I'm happy to help them because I'm just so grateful to be back to my old happy self again. Even now, I still say a little thank you to my guardian angel before and after every run.

How Beryl did it

Motivation tip: 'I have little motivational things I repeat to myself in my head, such as "Keep focused" and "When you've got the ball, you've got to run with it." They help stop me running out of steam when I'm finding it hard.'

Eating tip: 'Take one day of eating at a time. Don't worry about what you ate yesterday or what you're going to eat tomorrow, just concentrate on getting today right.'

'SURVIVING CANCER MEANS I APPRECIATE EVERY RUN'

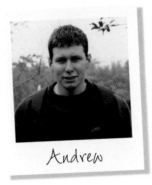

Andrew

After undergoing chemotherapy for testicular cancer at the age of 18, ANDREW SHIPPEY, from Leeds, was unable even to walk. But running got him back on his feet – and enabled him to raise an astounding half a million pounds for research into fighting cancer

❝ Seven years ago, testicular cancer tore a big hole in my life. I was just your average 18-year-old when I was diagnosed and told I had a 50/50 chance of survival. But I did survive, and four years later I triumphantly finished the Great North Run half-marathon, feeling absolutely amazing.

Most people watching the race that day wouldn't have guessed how hard I had to fight to get there, and that I had tens of thousands of people supporting me and resting their hopes on me. And even I didn't know that by crossing that finish line, I'd raised more than £500,000 to fund research into the disease that nearly killed me. Through running I regained my fitness and transformed a terrible situation into a life-affirming one.

shocked and devastated
Before I developed cancer, I was very active – I was a regular runner and loved football. It was while I was

playing football during the Easter break at university that I first realised I was ill. I remember the date exactly: Tuesday, 8 April. I got a knock in the stomach and felt so sick that I threw up. In A&E, the doctors suspected I had a burst ulcer, but they conducted

'There was no way I was going to let cancer beat me – I had an unshakeable conviction I was going to get better'

further tests just to be sure. Things moved at lightning speed after that: on 10 April I was told I had cancer. Two days later, I was having chemotherapy.

The doctors waited for my mum and dad to arrive before they told me the bad news. I was devastated and shocked but felt I had to put on a brave face in front of them. Once they'd gone home, I kept thinking, 'You're 18 and you're dying,' and kept asking, 'Why me?'. But I woke up the next day with a completely different attitude. There was no way I was going to let cancer beat me, and I had an unshakeable conviction that I was going to get better. I kept telling

'I was told the cancer had spread to my liver and lungs and there was now only a 50/50 chance I'd survive'

myself that testicular cancer is 95% curable if it's caught early.

However, after my first chemo session, I was dealt another blow when I was told the cancer had spread to my liver and lungs and there was now only a 50/50 chance I'd survive. My dad was nearly in tears but I just laughed it off as I was 100% certain I was going to get better. The doctors suggested a high-dose chemotherapy that was so toxic they'd have to harvest stem cells from my blood to help replace all the healthy cells it would kill along with the cancerous ones.

The chemotherapy knocked me for six. I was hospitalised for five weeks, spent four days in intensive care and was so ill that I don't remember two weeks of that time. Afterwards, I had to have hours of physio to help me walk again as I'd been flat on my back for so long. I also had to have two operations.

joy and relief

I'll never forget the day I got the all-clear in October. I'd gone for a check-up after my operation and expected to be told I'd need one more dose of chemotherapy but the doctor told me it wouldn't be necessary. I wanted to jump up and kiss her! My mum was with me and when we got outside I

said, 'I told you I could do it!' I spent the rest of the day visiting my friends to tell them the good news before hitting the pub. I can't begin to describe the sore head I had the next day – but I didn't care!

starting over

I was determined from then on to get the most out of life every single day. As a first step, I set my sights on playing in a singles-versus-marrieds football match my club had organised, and started running to get fit for it. On my first run I got so carried away that I went way too far too soon and ended up aching like hell for several days afterwards. However, it felt great being able to do something I wanted to do for a change instead of having my whole life dictated to me as it had

'On my first run I got so carried away, I went way too far too soon and ached like hell afterwards'

been when I was in hospital.

I made it through the match and the following year I went back to university to complete my degree. I continued running and the following year decided to do the Great North Run in Newcastle upon Tyne. I thought I'd gain an enormous sense of achievement doing something like that: to beat cancer you have to be tough, which is exactly what you have to be to run 21K (13.1 miles). I found the race quite challenging, but then so did the friends I ran with. I had no difficulty keeping up with them and didn't seem to have been affected by my illness. That year and the next, I raised about £100 each time for Cancer Research UK and was really chuffed with that.

payback time

Then came a call from Cancer Research UK who said it was looking for someone to run the Great North Run, around whom it could base a big charity fundraising campaign. I readily agreed as I was really keen to give something back to them. I knew I owed my life to it – the high-dose chemo I'd been given had been developed with the help of one of its grants.

I had an awesome time on the day – the atmosphere at the start, when we lined up with a crowd of more than 30,000 people, was amazing. I ran with eight friends and we stuck together throughout, chatting, laughing and encouraging each other. It was much hotter than it had been in previous years and I was near to collapse not far from the end when a kind person in the crowd handed me a biscuit that gave me a huge sugar – and morale – boost. I knew I simply had to make it to the finish line as I had so much money riding on me – an astonishing £370,000! When I finally got to the end, I thought, 'The money's in the bank!'

amazing support

But the best was yet to come. Several weeks later, Cancer Research UK called to say that a mailshot it had sent out after the race had raised even more sponsorship and that my total was now a staggering £533,000. I was speechless and very touched that more than 32,000 people had sponsored me, including a pensioner who'd called Cancer Research UK to ask what my race number was. She said she and her friends in the old people's home wanted to be able to spot 'their boy' on the TV.

hope and glory

I think the reason people responded to my appeal was that it was a good hope story – perhaps they thought, 'He's a young kid, he's had cancer, and yet he's willing to run 13 miles. He got off his backside to do something amazing.' I think I helped them see that there's life after cancer.

I've been clear of cancer for more than six years now, and will carry on doing the Great North Run for charity every year, though I know my previous sponsorship total will take some beating! I owe a lot to running – being fit before I became ill played a major role in my recovery. Running helped me build myself up again. Now, every time I go for a run I'm celebrating being alive. **"**

How Andrew did it

Motivation tip: 'Raise money for charity but choose something you care passionately about so you'll feel you're letting people down if you don't finish the race.'

Training tip: 'Always build up gradually and don't drain your body by overdoing it. And don't forget to ease up on your training the week before a race.'

'I RAN THE LONDON MARATHON – WHILE IN PRISON'

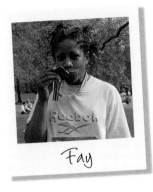

Fay

When FAY JOHNSON, 41, from London, went to prison for fraud, her self-esteem hit an all-time low. But being offered the chance to run the London Marathon while serving her sentence rebuilt her faith in herself and her abilities

" When I was sent to prison at HMP Downview, in Surrey, I found it incredibly hard to cope because everything was so different from the outside world. I had to leave behind my old life with my 14-year-old son and my partner, and face a four-year sentence inside. I started out in a tiny cell, with a toilet just a foot away from my bed and bars on the windows. Our doors were locked from 8pm until 8am, and the only thing I could do was sit in my cell and read my Bible. I didn't find it easy to get along with lots of the other prisoners and, although my faith helped me keep going, it was a truly terrible time.

We were allowed out of our cells during the day, so I started spending all my time at the prison gym. At 89kg (14st) and a size 18, I was incredibly unconfident, so I'd just sit on the exercise bike and pedal for hours. The PE officers noticed that I was going to the gym a lot and one, Linda Charles (whom everyone calls Charlie), offered me the chance to do a Community Sports Leader qualification, which I passed without any problem. All the exercise I had to do on the course also meant I slimmed down to about 67kg (10st 6lb). After that, Charlie offered me a job as a gym orderly and I was also moved into a nicer wing at the prison.

In early January one year the governor of the prison offered me a place in that year's London Marathon, raising money for a charity called The Hardman Trust, which helps

'I started my four-year sentence in a tiny cell, with a toilet just a foot from my bed and barred windows'

rehabilitate prisoners. My first thought was, 'You've asked the wrong person, I can't possibly do it.' I'd never been a runner, and didn't think I could even run to the end of the road. But Charlie stepped in and reminded me that I didn't have to win, just finish. She told me she was convinced I could do it, which made me feel it would be an insult to her judgement to tell her I couldn't. Thinking about it alone in my cell, I realised it was the first time in ages that something nice had happened to me, so I plucked up the courage to say yes.

'Three prison officers took it in turns to run on the treadmill beside me to help keep me motivated'

shaky start

My first run was only a couple of minutes on the prison treadmill. My legs couldn't keep up with the pace of the machine, even when it was going really slowly, but Charlie just told me she believed in me and said I had to get on with it. From then on, I started running almost every day, and after ten days I was ecstatic when I ran a whole mile without stopping. It never felt easy, though, because as soon as I improved, Charlie moved the goalposts again to make things harder. Nevertheless, I started looking forward to my runs and enjoying the company I had while I was running – Charlie organised prison officers to take it in turns to run on the treadmill beside me to keep me motivated. The first time I ran 14.4K (9 miles), three officers each did 5K (3-mile) stints on the treadmill next to mine.

mind games

After that, I was allowed outside to start running round the prison's Astroturf football pitch. By the end of February, I managed the magic total of 21K (13.1 miles) – a half-marathon – by running 93 laps. It was quite a challenge running round and round in circles, and to help me keep count of the laps I'd think about counting objects – like two apples to remind me I was on lap two – and so on. Running became like an escape for me, and despite being in prison, I felt a sense of freedom at being able to go off into my own thoughts. Even though I was feeling fitter, I still found it difficult to believe the marathon was really going to happen – it seemed like part of the outside world that I didn't live in any more.

running free

Eight weeks before the marathon, I was allowed out of prison so Charlie could take me to buy trainers for the race. She had to get a special licence for the outing, but although she had to stay close by me, she didn't have to handcuff me. It was a real treat to see all the shops again. I wanted to go

'After two months, I managed to do a half-marathon – by running 93 laps round the prison's football pitch'

window shopping, but of course Charlie wouldn't let me!

After that, Charlie also applied to be able to take me running outside the prison. It felt very different running on the hard concrete instead of a soft treadmill or Astroturf, but it was wonderful to see things such as houses and gardens, which I hadn't seen for such a long time. Charlie also asked the prison kitchen to prepare pasta dishes for me and ordered bananas and sports drinks specially for me. All the other inmates and prison officers were very supportive of me as well.

The night before the marathon, I lay in my cell and thought about how proud I was that Charlie and the rest of the prison had put their trust in me, and how I didn't want to let them down. I also knew that a huge amount of my self-esteem rested on my getting round the marathon course.

the big day
On the morning of the marathon, I got up at 3am because I was so afraid of oversleeping. I had a big breakfast and set off really early with Charlie, heading for the start in Greenwich. Standing on the start line, I felt a lot more excited and nervous than I'd expected. I was allowed to run on my own, and just meet Charlie at the finish line. Rather than chatting to people, I kept my head down and tried to stay focused, but I really loved seeing all the London sights again, and also the way all the children in the crowd put their hands up to clap my hand as I ran by. I saw Charlie, who kept popping up at different points, and also met up with my partner and son at the finish line. I was surprised that even though it had taken me more than six hours to run the race, there were still huge crowds cheering us on, and I know my son was totally amazed to see me do something so sporty! I amazed myself, too, and now that it's all over, I still can't quite believe I did

it. I think if I didn't have my medal to prove it, it would feel like a dream.

future hopes
What the marathon taught me is that if someone believes in you enough to offer a helping hand, you can achieve the unthinkable. I'm up for parole soon and can finally see a future for myself outside prison. Thanks to the running and the fitness course I did, I now have the confidence and ambition to set up my own fitness business, working with obese children.

As a thank you, I want to donate my marathon medal to Charlie as she put in as much hard work as I did! I know she was incredibly proud because she's never trained someone to run a marathon before. It's also a way of thanking her for trusting me, and giving me a chance to prove that I could do it. I would love it to hang in the prison gym and inspire other prisoners to do a marathon. I hope I've paved the way for them to have a go, too – and that they get just as much out of it as I did. 99

How Fay did it
Motivation tip: 'I only ever thought of my short-term goals. If Charlie set me a task, I always achieved it as I never wanted to come back and admit I couldn't do it.'
Eating tip: 'I started eating porridge for breakfast when I began training for the marathon, and I still have it now. It's really filling and satisfying but also low in calories.'

'NO ONE KNEW WHETHER I'D SURVIVE MY FALL'

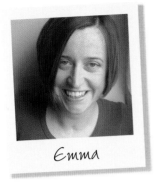

Emma

A terrible accident left EMMA DOBINSON, 30, from London, in a coma and with a serious brain injury. Now, four years on, she's made an amazing recovery, using running, and one special race, as her lifeline

❝ Before I had my accident, I was really sporty, and used to run regularly. Now, four years down the line, running has helped me claw my way back to feeling fit and healthy again. It took a lot of courage for me to dare to try running after what I'd been through, but I'm so glad I did because it really helped me recover both physically and emotionally.

The accident happened at about 1.30am one Monday morning. I was returning home in a taxi after a night out with friends, when I'd drunk far too much. I was also feeling absolutely shattered because I'd been really busy at work. The taxi driver said later that when he dropped me off, I didn't go into my house but set off down the road. I have no idea where I was going or why – in fact, I don't know anything about the lead-up to the accident except what I've since been told, because it wiped out part of my memory. I ended up at a block of nearby flats, where I fell about 4.5m (15ft) over the edge of the first-floor walkway. About four hours later, a stranger found me lying on the ground, bleeding heavily with a huge gash in my head and a mangled left arm.

fighting for survival

I stayed in a coma for nearly two weeks. I had seriously injured my brain and the doctors had to remove a part of my skull to help reduce the pressure that had built up. They also had to

'A stranger found me lying on the ground, bleeding heavily with a huge gash in my head'

insert long metal screws into my arm to repair my shattered elbow. When I first came round, I couldn't speak, and people had to interpret what I wanted from the expressions in my eyes and blinking alone. The whole thing was very traumatic for everyone – the police opened an investigation to try to find out whether anyone else had been involved or tried to hurt me, and also questioned me over whether I might have been trying deliberately to harm myself. They decided no one else was involved, but I still have to live with the uncertainty of not knowing exactly what happened or why.

My short-term memory was very badly affected by the fall and, once I started talking again, I'd get my words jumbled up (I'd tell my visitors to sit on the toilet, when I was pointing at a chair). I was also totally exhausted and had to spend hours sleeping. After four months in hospital, I was finally allowed to go back home, and that's when exercise started to play a role in my recovery. Having to cope with the outside world, and even silly things such as reading bank statements, felt like a lot to handle, and I was very upset because my arm wouldn't work

'I'd work out wearing a brightly coloured headscarf to hide my massive bald patch and scar'

properly. I moved back home so my parents could care for me, but this meant giving up a lot of independence. Exercise allowed me to feel that I was at least helping myself.

first steps
I started with really gentle walking and cycling once a week at my local gym – I had to avoid impact exercise so my brain wouldn't pulsate too much. I'd work out wearing a brightly coloured headscarf because I had a massive bald patch, a huge scar and a bulging shape to my head that wasn't very attractive! Even though it was strange

to find the exercise so tiring, I stuck at it and was so proud when after a while I was upgraded to going to the gym twice a week.

I was beginning to regain some of my old strength when my friend Bally

'There was an adrenaline buzz in the air – the race seemed to mean so much to everyone there'

told me about the Flora Light Challenge For Women, a 5K (3-mile) race that takes place in Hyde Park in London every year. I became determined to walk the race with her because I needed a goal and wanted to prove that I was getting fitter and healthier again.

The race and the walking I was doing to prepare for it became my main aim in life, and the day more than lived up to my expectations. The thousands of people taking part and the amount of support we got from the crowds were just amazing. There was a tangible adrenaline buzz in the air and the race seemed to mean so much to everyone there.

Bally and I speed-walked round the course chatting the whole way, and even finished in front of some of the runners, watched proudly by my mum, dad and Bally's boyfriend. I was thrilled to collect my medal and, as I handed over the £1,000 cheque I'd raised for charity to my consultant, he was amazed at how well I'd done. That race gave me support, motivation and self-belief. I was even able to start working again as a film researcher because I'd regained so much confidence. It very quickly became my goal to work up to running the race the following year, and I felt full of hope that I'd be able to keep on improving.

learning to run again

Two years on from my accident, I had to have another big operation to replace the missing piece of my skull, and had to take barbiturates to prevent me from having fits, which left me feeling pretty lethargic and awful. A few months later, I was given the all-clear to go running for the first time since I'd had my accident, and I decided I'd start training so I could do the Flora Light Challenge For Women again. The first outing was pretty nerve-wracking. I set off very gently on my own, following a walk/run programme and thinking, 'I hope nothing goes ker-plunk in my head and that bits of my brain don't explode!' I was worried about whether my feet were hitting the ground too hard and sending shockwaves to my brain.

I got a real confidence boost from finding I was fitter than I'd expected, and the longer I was able to run for, the more capable I started to feel. At times I'd be running along wanting to shout out to people, 'Look at me, I can do it, I'm really running!' And although it was hard to motivate myself sometimes as the barbiturates I was taking made me feel apathetic, once I got myself outside, running really helped counteract their effect.

running with a secret

I completed my second Flora Light Challenge For Women with Bally and my sister in about 30 minutes, and felt incredibly proud of my time. Once

again, it was an amazing experience, this time because my sister did it with me, and I realised how much my fitness and health had improved since the previous year. I also loved the fact that anyone watching us run wouldn't have known what had happened to me. I think of my accident as my little secret, unless I choose to tell people about it.

yearly milestone

The following year I took part again (although I had to walk as I'd injured a ligament) and I'm planning to keep on running the race every year. It's become a milestone on the road to recovery for me, and I even think of it as my own race because it means so much to me. I'm keen to keep getting faster, too!

When I look round and realise lots of people are afraid to try running, I'm so grateful that I dared to give it another go. Taking part in the race has shown me that I can achieve anything I want to if I set my mind to it. 99

How Emma did it

Motivation tip: 'On days when I struggled to motivate myself, I would just try to remember how much running helped me escape from my stresses and frustrations and how much better I felt after I'd run.'

Training tip: 'I followed a walk/run programme, which was a great way back into running. It's really important to take things slowly at first.'

'I WANTED TO RUN SO BADLY, I RAN ON CRUTCHES'

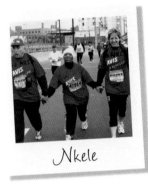

Nkele

Having only one leg wasn't going to stop NKELE MOSIANE, 38 (centre), from fulfilling her childhood dream of running. That's why this South African from Johannesburg joined a running club and ran three marathons – on crutches

❝ I come from South Africa and in my culture it's traditional to name your child after something you've seen or experienced when giving birth. My name, Nkele, means 'tears' and I've often wondered why my mother called me this. Were they tears of joy at the birth of her first daughter or tears of sorrow because I was born disabled? I don't know why, but I never plucked up the courage to ask her – I like to think it was the former.

I was born with a twisted left foot that had two extra toes and I didn't have a tibia in my left leg so, when I was five, my leg was amputated at the knee. At the age of six, I was fitted with a very crude wood, steel and rubber artificial limb, which enabled me to walk with the aid of crutches. I hated using crutches so I was really pleased when I got my first proper artificial leg at the age of nine, which meant I could walk unsupported.

I found it really difficult being disabled as the other children at my school called me names like 'cripple'. Back then, I would never have dreamed that one day I'd have run five marathons and have a big collection of

'I found it hard being disabled as the other children at my school called me names like "cripple"'

more than thirty running medals hanging up proudly in my hallway!

raring to go
One April, when I was working at the Self Help Centre For Paraplegics in Soweto, near Johannesburg, the Achilles Track Club [an organisation that aims to encourage disabled people to participate in long-distance running] called and told me it was recruiting members for the new running club it was starting. When I was a schoolgirl, I used to love watching my friends do athletics and yearned to be able to join them. I really hated having to sit on the sidelines watching them run. So when I got the call, I thought to

myself, 'At last, this is my chance, I'll give it a try,' and went along to a local sports field with two other women who'd also had their legs amputated, to see if I'd be able to do it. I'd never run so much as a step before so I found running very difficult. My artificial leg was so heavy that I was forced to use crutches, and at first I could only walk.

At every training session I was always the last person to finish, but I persevered because I just loved doing it so much. We started out doing 2K

'I loved running but doing it with crutches was tough as I got really painful blisters on my hands'

(just over a mile) and it took me 90 minutes to finish. Eventually, I decided to remove my artificial leg as it was holding me back, and just use crutches. Running with crutches was tough as I got really painful blisters on my hands. I developed a style of running that I call the double hop – I'd place both crutches a little way ahead of me and then swing my right foot and left stump through. It was a strange way to run!

crowd support

As an incentive, we entered a 32K (20-mile) race in February the following year. I thoroughly enjoyed it because of all the support I got from the runners and spectators. Their words of encouragement helped me get where I wanted to be – the finish. I got cramp in my foot and thigh and blisters on my hands and foot during the race, but I was elated when I'd done it. I

kept looking at my medal and thinking, 'Most able-bodied people don't have a medal, but now I do!'

spills and thrills

Soon after that first race, I was incredibly excited to be asked whether I'd like to be sponsored by the New York Achilles Track Club to run the New York City Marathon. I had high hopes but that marathon was a real struggle. I was just so nervous, and it was raining and freezing cold. I fell over twice because my crutches slipped on the wet road, but I gritted my teeth and kept going. I told myself there was no way I could fly all the way from South Africa to America and not finish.

I ran for 750m (½ mile), then walked for 750m, until the final 8K (5 miles), when I ran all the way. I was accompanied by two fantastic American guides who made sure I had everything I needed (they even gave me a roadside massage when I got cramp!). Listening to them and telling them what it's like to live in South

'I fell over twice because my crutches slipped on the wet road, but I gritted my teeth and kept going'

Africa helped distract me from the blisters on my hands. The crowd were also amazing – they kept shouting, 'Go! Go! You're almost there!' I loved that crowd because they encouraged me so much. It took me 12 hours and 12 minutes to finish that day, and I felt exhausted but also very proud of what I'd achieved.

big surprise!

I ended up running the New York City Marathon five times in total, and after I'd completed the third one, I was given a big surprise. I'd been promised a new, lightweight artificial leg before by the New York Achilles Track Club, but each time I'd been bumped on to the waiting list as there'd been other runners whose need was greater than mine. But this time, I was finally given one that was light enough to run with. I was overjoyed as it was really expensive and there was no way I could have afforded to buy such a sophisticated leg myself. At last, I could ditch the crutches and run almost normally – even though I had a slight limp, I felt an incredible sense of freedom. I had to get used to the new leg, which was very painful to use in the beginning. On the places where my stump put pressure on it, I got terrible blisters, but I didn't let that put me off.

I've since run two other New York City Marathons with my new leg, and I've got faster each time. My current personal best time is 8:45 and my next goal is to run it in under eight hours. Along the way, I've also run more than thirty races.

proud moments

Running has made me what I am – before I used to obsess about my problems but now I just focus on how I'm going to run my next race. It's given me self-belief and confidence: I no longer see myself as physically challenged, but instead see myself as physically challenging as I'm constantly challenging myself.

I love encouraging others to run, too. When my friends say they also want to take up running, I say, 'Come along and we'll see what you can do.' I've now helped train the two women who did the New York City Marathon with me – when we all finished, I felt I'd done a really good job. What I'm most proud of, however, is the way I've inspired my daughter. She wasn't a runner, but after she had seen me enter a few races it prompted her to join a running club. Her name is Mapule,

> 'I'm not physically challenged… I see myself as physically challenging as I'm constantly challenging myself'

which means 'rain', because it was raining when she was born. It's amusing to think that the only thing I don't like about running is doing it when it's raining!

How Nkele did it

Motivation tip: 'If you're tempted to skip a training session, ask yourself, "What will I be doing instead?" You'll soon realise that unless you've got really good alternative plans, you'll feel guilty about not going and a lot better if you do.'

Eating tip: 'To give you energy during a run, eat small amounts of foods like sweets, chocolate and bananas.'

'I'VE DONE 30 MARATHONS – SINCE THE AGE OF 71!'

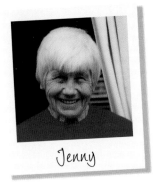

Jenny

JENNY WOOD ALLEN, 92, is an unstoppable great grandmother from Dundee, Scotland, who has run her way to a world record and well and truly proved that pensioners aren't past it

❝ When I'm asked why I took up marathon running at the age of 71, I always reply, 'For the money!' In the 30 marathons I ran until I retired from the sport aged 90, I raised more than £36,000 for various charities.

As a child, I didn't do anything vaguely athletic except play. I never did sports at school either as I was so clumsy – the knees of the long, black stockings we wore in those days were always full of holes as I kept falling over. At the age of 19, I bought a bike, inspired by my elder brother, who was a keen cyclist. The only catch was, I didn't have a clue how to ride it, so I'd go out early every Sunday morning and practise. I fell off countless times but was glad I persevered as I soon became hooked.

I think I must have had a latent competitive streak because I started competing in time trials, and by the early 1930s I was the fastest female road time-trial cyclist in Scotland. I kept on cycling with my husband, Roy, until 1962, when he was forced to give up cycling for medical reasons, and then for 20 years I didn't do any vigorous exercise at all.

daring to do it

The turning point came when I was aged 71 and, as a city councillor, was helping organise the inaugural Dundee Marathon. I don't know what came over me that day but I

'My son hooted with laughter when I told him I'd decided to enter my first marathon aged 71'

impulsively decided to enter, mainly to help the Dundee Sports Association for the Disabled raise funds for a specially adapted minibus. The only running I'd ever done was at Sunday School picnics, when I'd usually come dead last. When I told my son, he hooted with laughter and said, 'Mum, you never run, except for the bus, and even then you miss it!'

Five months before the race in April 1983, I donned my slacks, anorak and walking shoes and got down to serious training. I felt really self-conscious as there weren't many other runners out on the roads at that time – and there certainly weren't any with white hair and wrinkles! – so I'd take a shopping bag along with me and pretend I was in a hurry to get to the shops. I didn't stick to a particular programme, but each day I found I was able to go

'I felt self-conscious when training, so I'd take a shopping bag and pretend I was in a hurry to get to the shops'

farther. I trained alone as I don't think anyone in my family wanted to be blamed for encouraging me!

agony and ecstasy

Finally, marathon day dawned and I set off, full of trepidation. The longest run I'd done in training had been a half-marathon, so when I got halfway and felt my legs start to ache, I told them sternly, "Don't seize up!' and just kept on going, hoping they'd hold out for the next 21K (13.1 miles).

When I crossed the finish line in 5 hours and 34 minutes I felt elation along with an overwhelming sense of relief. I managed to raise £1,000, a considerable sum in those days. My family and friends were all really pleased for me, but they didn't make too much of a fuss of me – I think they wanted to keep my feet on the ground! Even though I couldn't walk down stairs for days afterwards, after that first marathon I was bitten by the marathon bug and ran about

two marathons a year for 19 years from then on, training pretty much all year-round.

camaraderie and inspiration

What I like most about running is that it's something that enables me to stop worrying about trivial things and helps me put things in perspective. When my husband died 11 years ago, I couldn't sleep, but I got up the next day and went for a run and felt a lot calmer. I even went out running on the morning of his funeral. It's also been great for my figure – I went from a size 14/16 to a 12 and lost 10.5kg (1st 9lb).

The great sense of camaraderie I feel with other runners is what kept me running marathon after marathon. It's lovely being surrounded by so many people with the same goal. It's also wonderful hearing the crowd egging me on. My daughter-in-law gave me the white canvas hat with my name on it that I always wear, because she felt the crowd would cheer me on even

'At times, the roar of the crowd cheering me on is so loud it sounds as if I'm at Wembley stadium!'

more if they knew my name – and she was right. At times, the roar is so loud it sounds as if I'm at Wembley stadium!

Over the years, I've come across many truly inspirational runners. In particular, I remember one young man whose courage really impressed me. He'd been devastated when he'd been diagnosed with motor neurone disease, and entered the Flora London Marathon as he knew it was his last chance to run it. When I met him at a press conference a few days before the race, he was already on crutches, but he nonetheless made it to the finish. A couple of weeks later he was confined to a wheelchair.

I'm often told that I've inspired a lot of people to take up running, but I've noticed I'm inspiring in another way, too. When I pass younger runners who are walking during a race, it's amusing to see how they suddenly start running again!

world record

Most of the time I'm not competing against other runners, I simply want to do a respectable time. But the highlight of my racing career was running the Dundee Marathon aged 74. I ran it in 4:21, and when I finished I couldn't believe my eyes and thought the clock had stopped. A few days later, however, I was even more amazed when a reporter called to tell me I'd broken the previous world record for a woman over 70 by 20 minutes.

90 not out

I've certainly had some lows, too. At the 30K (19-mile) mark in one London Marathon, someone ran into the back of me, sending me sprawling. The ambulance crew I hobbled over to insisted that I stop running as they said they were packing up and there might not be an ambulance if I needed one later in the race. Reluctantly, I agreed to throw in the towel – but it was really galling to have done 30K (19 miles) and not finish.

I did my last marathon at the age of 90 in London – I walked it in 11 hours and 34 minutes. My knees and thighs were suffering, but I was determined to finish. I've now given up doing marathons as the training takes up so much time, but I continue to run shorter distances.

young at heart

Many people have asked me why I think I've been able to run so many marathons while other pensioners would blanch at the thought. The answer's easy – other pensioners simply don't *want* to run marathons! I firmly believe that determination is the secret of my success. I don't think of myself as old – I'm simply older. And I think my running has helped me prove that I'm not just an old dear.

Throughout my running career, dozens of people have come up to me and said, 'You're wonderful.' But I don't think I'm wonderful – I just feel I want to join in with the young ones and not be left out. **99**

How Jenny did it

Motivation tip: 'The hardest step is the one over your doorstep, so before you start, try to picture the glow of satisfaction you'll feel once you've finished. And don't forget to enjoy yourself!'
Eating tip: 'Before all my marathons, I always breakfast on two helpings of Complan, a meal-replacement powder that you mix with milk. It's great if you can't face solid food first thing in the morning.'

'I'M BLIND BUT I DO THINGS SIGHTED RUNNERS CAN'T'

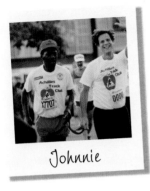

Johnnie

JOHNNIE DEMAS (far left), 56, from Johannesburg, South Africa, lost his sight in a vicious gang attack more than thirty years ago. Yet 11 years later, he took his first tentative steps as a blind runner, holding one end of a handkerchief while a sighted runner held the other...

❝ I've been blind for more than thirty years. I live in Johannesburg, which can be a very violent city, and my life changed for ever one day in November 1974, when, aged 26, I was attacked by a gang, who mistook me for someone else. I suffered multiple stab wounds and my skull was fractured by a brick. After the attack, I had brain surgery and was unconscious for 45 days. The doctors didn't think I'd survive and feared I'd be brain damaged. Waking up from that coma was terrible – when I found that all I could see was blackness, I knew I'd gone blind, and that I'd be blind for life. I felt rage at the gang for doing such a thing to me and I also felt helpless as there was nothing I could do about it.

big adjustment
It truly was the hardest time in my life. I felt so miserable and found adjusting to being blind very difficult. I felt I had no future because, as a bricklayer, there was no way I could continue with my job. I was single at the time but I thank God for my family, who helped me through.

life-changing moment
For six years I was unable to work and I lived off a disability pension, but then I managed to get a job glueing handles into paper carrier bags at the Services for the Blind and Visually

'When I woke up from the coma, all I could see was blackness and I knew I'd be blind for life'

Handicapped organisation. It didn't pay very much but I enjoyed it. I began to feel less depressed because I met other people who'd also once been able to see but were now blind. Before that I'd thought I was the only person in the world that this had happened to.

My life changed again one day when Denis Tabakin, who works for the Achilles Track Club [an organisation that aims to encourage disabled people to participate in long-distance running], came to my workplace and gave a talk about running. He said it was possible for blind people to run by

'In the beginning it was hard learning to put my total trust in my guide but I learnt to just run in faith'

holding on to one end of a handkerchief while a sighted person held the other. Quite a few of us were tempted to give running a go, and so, accompanied by Denis and two social workers, we went off to try it out.

In the beginning I found running really scary as I was terrified of smacking into a lamp-post or tree. It was hard learning to put my total trust in my guide. Eventually, however, I got used to it – I learnt not to worry about where I was putting my feet and just run in faith. I found my hearing became more acute as I had to listen out for traffic and other runners, and I also began to 'read' the road with my feet.

Over several weeks we built up to doing 5K (3 miles) and then we entered an 8K (5-mile) fun run. It was my first race and I really enjoyed it. When I won a bottle of Scotch whisky in the prize draw, I thought, 'I'll definitely be back for more!'

racing ahead

Our group of eight runners eventually joined the Rocky Road Runners Club, which had lots of members willing to be guides, and I'm a member to this

day. I gradually increased the distances I was running and then began to wonder whether I'd be able to do the Johannesburg Marathon. I trained really hard and did it in 4:24. After that, I began to think of myself as a real runner and became totally hooked on running! Instead of spending my weekends moping around the house feeling sorry for myself, I entered races most Sundays, met lots of new people and made new friends.

Soon, I realised marathons weren't enough and I set my sights on the Comrades ultra-marathon, an 89K (55.6-mile) race. With my guide, Richard Shakenovsky, I managed to do it in 10:29. It never crossed my mind that we wouldn't finish and I was positive the whole time. You have to be mentally strong to tackle a distance as long as Comrades. Finishing felt so great – I simply couldn't quite believe

'It felt great finishing the Comrades ultra-marathon – I simply couldn't quite believe I'd run 89K'

I'd run 89K. I've run it every year since and love doing it – it's just a big fun day out for me.

That year was also memorable in another way because I married my wife, Ida, whom I'd met at work. She's blind, too, and even though she's not a runner herself, she's really proud of what I've achieved. We have two children, Lorimee and Richard, who's named after my first guide. I manage to combine running with family life by running 9K (5.6 miles) before work three times a week. I meet my running partner, Gerald Fox, at 5.45am and we run from there to work. On Sundays I go for a longer run.

great guides

I've had several guides (we call them pilots!) over the years and they've all become close friends. We take turns setting the pace, which can be frustrating at times, and if one of us needs the loo, the other simply has to wait for him. I'm not a talkative person but I like running with a guide, especially a chatty one, because it helps keep my mind off how far we have to go. My guide tells me how the other runners are doing and describes the scenery so I can imagine what it looks like and appreciate it, too. He also warns me of any obstacles and tells me if there's a hill ahead. But if he loses concentration, it can have disastrous consequences. One year, when I was running the Two Oceans Marathon in Cape Town, my guide started chatting to some other runners just as we passed a water table. I slipped on the discarded cups and injured my knees really badly. It didn't stop me finishing, but he felt terribly guilty afterwards.

marathon man

Why do I love running? Well, it makes me feel good and has helped me have a better self-image. I used to be overweight but I've lost 8kg (1st 4lb) and look great. I'm also proud of all my achievements and think it's wonderful that I can do something that many sighted runners haven't done. One such achievement was doing the

Golden Reef 100 Miler (160K), which I ran to raise funds for a charity that cares for abused and HIV-positive children. I ran most of the way but walked up the hills and it took me 22 hours and 58 minutes! So far, I've done 40 marathons and 16 consecutive Comrades, a record for a blind runner, and my goal is to run 20. When other runners call me 'The Marathon Man' or say, 'Here's the Comrades King!,' it feels fantastic.

whole new world

Running has totally transformed my life. I've made life-long friends with my guides and it even helped me get the job I have now as I met my current running partner and boss, Gerald, through the Rocky Road Runners.

I wonder if I'd be a runner today if I hadn't been blinded. Running has opened up a whole new world for me. It's helped me feel that I'm just as good as anyone else – it's just that I can't see. I love it when fellow runners say to me, "You're an amazing man – you've got all the excuses in the world not to run but you still do it. 99

How Johnnie did it

Motivation tip: 'Try to do your run first thing to make sure you don't get distracted by other commitments during the day.'
Training tip: 'Run with a friend because you can't let them down. I meet my partner at a certain place each time and I know I can't let him stand there and not turn up!'

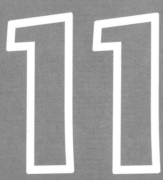

Kick off your trainers, put your feet up and pour yourself a drink – it's time to celebrate just how far you've come…

11
get celebrating

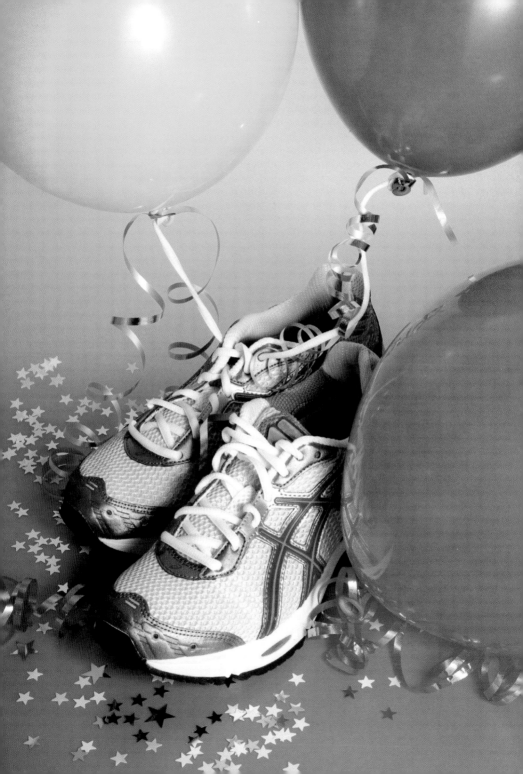

Celebrate yourself

Hurrah – you've almost reached the end of this book, and you've come a long way, which is why we've decided to wind things up with a pause for celebration. So stop for a minute, and just think about where you started from – feeling daunted, bored or just plain scared by running – and how you're feeling now – hopefully really fit and full of enthusiasm. Even if you've yet to run a single step, we hope you're feeling fired up and ready to go, and you've learnt to think of this book as your new best friend who'll keep supporting you and inspiring you along the way. Never pass up a chance to celebrate your successes, however small: in the words of American author and stress coach Loretta LaRoche, 'Life is short, so wear your party pants!'

Celebrate running

Going into this project, we both thought we knew all about running – not necessarily the technical stuff, but we certainly thought we knew exactly how to do it and how it makes you feel. But now, thanks to writing this book, we've learnt to celebrate running for so many more things. Whenever we've been closeted away writing chapters and the ideas wouldn't flow, we'd get up and go for a run, returning to our computers with loads of inspiration. Then there are all the new expert tips and advice we've road-tested that have given us new cause for celebration. Every time someone shared a brilliant idea, we couldn't wait to go out and try it for ourselves – from the Rope Trick you use to get up hills (page 127) to clever ways to relax and distract yourself when you're running (pages 134 and 135).

Celebrate others

Most of all, though, we wanted to use this book to help celebrate the hundreds of runners who've done the most amazing things. At every turn, we've met and interviewed incredibly inspiring people who've all given up their time to share their stories for this book. From visiting Fay Johnson in prison and being allowed into her world for a couple of hours (page 187) to making transcontinental calls to one-legged runner Catherine Mokwena in South Africa on a phoneline that cut out 19 times (pages 44 and 209), every interview has been a voyage of discovery! It's time for you to celebrate other runners, too – here's a final list to help you do it...

MY TO-DO LIST

✔ Go and cheer at a race.

✔ Go and teach someone else to run – it's a gift that will last a lifetime.

✔ Go and smile at every other runner you pass in the park.

✔ Go and offer to run with someone who needs a motivation boost.

✔ Go and share this book.

✔ Go and round up a group of friends and run barefoot on a sandy beach – nothing beats it.

✔ Go enjoy.

✔ Just go!

We've done our bit and now it's *your* turn to get writing. Use the Ultimate Six-Month Running Diary to diarise and analyse every run. Good luck – and keep on running!

12

get scribbling

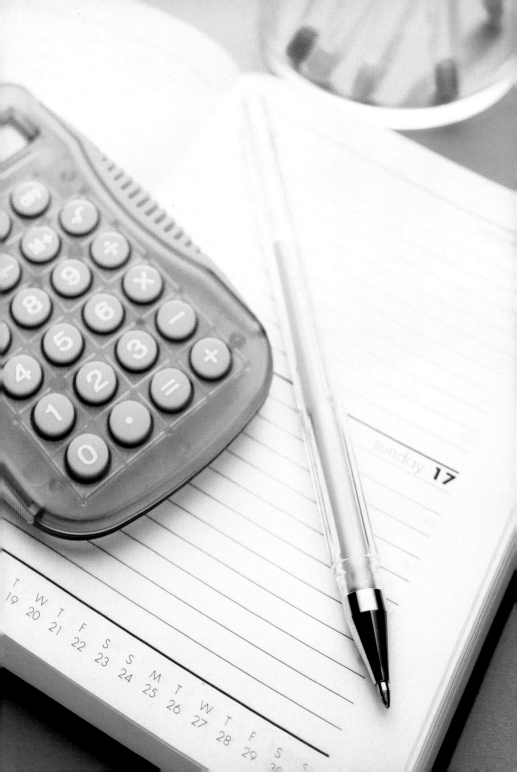

Your ultimate six-month running diary

Nothing's more satisfying than looking back on your training to see how far you've come. Each day you'll be making small, almost invisible improvements, until one day you'll wake up and realise that goals you once thought were impossible (running three times a week, running 5km/ 3 miles in under 30 minutes or even running a marathon) are either within reach or already ticked off on your 'Been there, done that' list.

Each time you go for a run, fill in the running diary on the pages that follow – and then review your progress regularly to see whether you can spot anything that will help you get even better, and adjust your training accordingly. So, for example, if you always have Euphoric runs on grass but Hellish ones on the treadmill, schedule more runs in the sun. (If you've forgotten exactly what those funky little Mood-O-Meter symbols mean, turn back to page 72 for the lowdown.)

Here's how to fill in the running diary – use whichever categories are useful to you, and feel free to ignore the rest!

⭐ **Date** Write down the date of when you did your session.

⭐ **Time** Write down how long you went out running for.

⭐ **Distance** (optional) If you know it, write down how far you ran in kilometres or miles.

⭐ **Type of run** Did you do an ordinary run or did you do some speed-training (such as intervals)?

⭐ **Where I ran** Write down whether you ran on a track, road, grass, pavement, trail or treadmill (if you ran on a treadmill, make a note of the incline and speed you ran at).

⭐ **Mood before/during/after** Simply draw the facial expression that best applies to you on the icons provided. Use the key at the top of the page to remind you of the options.

😖 Hellish   😐 Indifferent   😕 Up and down   🙂 Good   😊 EUPHORIC!

Date	Time	Distance	Type of run	Where I ran	Mood before	Mood during	Mood after
Mon							
Tues							
Weds							
Thurs							
Fri							
Sat							
Sun							

Mon							
Tues							
Weds							
Thurs							
Fri							
Sat							
Sun							

❝ It's not about being first or last, it's about having the courage to finish the race. ❞

Catherine Mokwena, administrator

😧 **Hellish**　😐 **Indifferent**　😬 **Up and down**　🙂 **Good**　😃 **EUPHORIC!**

Date	Time	Distance	Type of run	Where I ran	Mood before	Mood during	Mood after
Mon					😊	😊	😊
Tues					😊	😊	😊
Weds					😊	😊	😊
Thurs					😊	😊	😊
Fri					😊	😊	😊
Sat					😊	😊	😊
Sun					😊	😊	😊

Mon					😊	😊	😊
Tues					😊	😊	😊
Weds					😊	😊	😊
Thurs					😊	😊	😊
Fri					😊	😊	😊
Sat					😊	😊	😊
Sun					😊	😊	😊

> 66 Be your own hero, it's cheaper than a movie ticket. 99
>
> Doug Horton, science-fiction author

☹ **Hellish** 😐 **Indifferent** 😕 **Up and down** 😊 **Good** 😄 **EUPHORIC!**

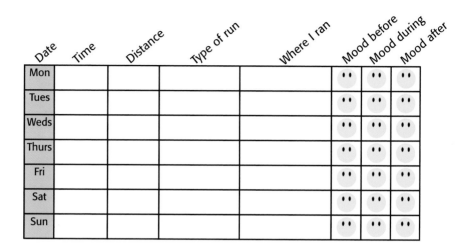

Date	Time	Distance	Type of run	Where I ran	Mood before	Mood during	Mood after
Mon							
Tues							
Weds							
Thurs							
Fri							
Sat							
Sun							

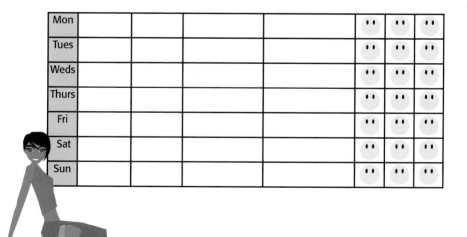

Mon							
Tues							
Weds							
Thurs							
Fri							
Sat							
Sun							

> **❝ All things excellent are as difficult as they are rare. ❞**
>
> Benedict de Spinoza, philosopher

☹ **Hellish** 😐 **Indifferent** 🙂 **Up and down** 😊 **Good** 😃 **EUPHORIC!**

Date	Time	Distance	Type of run	Where I ran	Mood before	Mood during	Mood after
Mon							
Tues							
Weds							
Thurs							
Fri							
Sat							
Sun							

Mon							
Tues							
Weds							
Thurs							
Fri							
Sat							
Sun							

> 66 The best preparation for tomorrow
> is doing your best today. 99
>
> Henry Jackson Brown Jr, writer

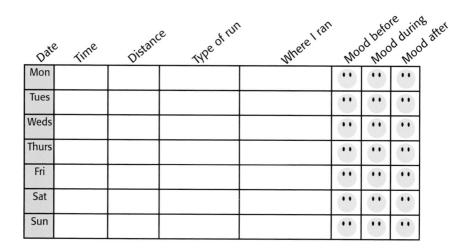

☹ **Hellish**　😐 **Indifferent**　😕 **Up and down**　🙂 **Good**　😃 **EUPHORIC!**

Date	Time	Distance	Type of run	Where I ran	Mood before	Mood during	Mood after
Mon					🙂	🙂	🙂
Tues					🙂	🙂	🙂
Weds					🙂	🙂	🙂
Thurs					🙂	🙂	🙂
Fri					🙂	🙂	🙂
Sat					🙂	🙂	🙂
Sun					🙂	🙂	🙂

Mon					🙂	🙂	🙂
Tues					🙂	🙂	🙂
Weds					🙂	🙂	🙂
Thurs					🙂	🙂	🙂
Fri					🙂	🙂	🙂
Sat					🙂	🙂	🙂
Sun					🙂	🙂	🙂

> 66 We can't all be heroes, because somebody has to sit on the curb and clap as they go by. 99
>
> Will Rogers, writer

Date	Time	Distance	Type of run	Where I ran	Mood before	Mood during	Mood after
Mon					🙂	🙂	🙂
Tues					🙂	🙂	🙂
Weds					🙂	🙂	🙂
Thurs					🙂	🙂	🙂
Fri					🙂	🙂	🙂
Sat					🙂	🙂	🙂
Sun					🙂	🙂	🙂

Mon					🙂	🙂	🙂
Tues					🙂	🙂	🙂
Weds					🙂	🙂	🙂
Thurs					🙂	🙂	🙂
Fri					🙂	🙂	🙂
Sat					🙂	🙂	🙂
Sun					🙂	🙂	🙂

> 66 Everyone runs the same distance in a race – if you look at the runners at the back, they're trying just as hard as those at the front – it's just that some people can go faster than others. 99
>
> Pippa Major, e-commerce development manager

😞 **Hellish**   😐 **Indifferent**   😊 **Up and down**   🙂 **Good**   😄 **EUPHORIC!**

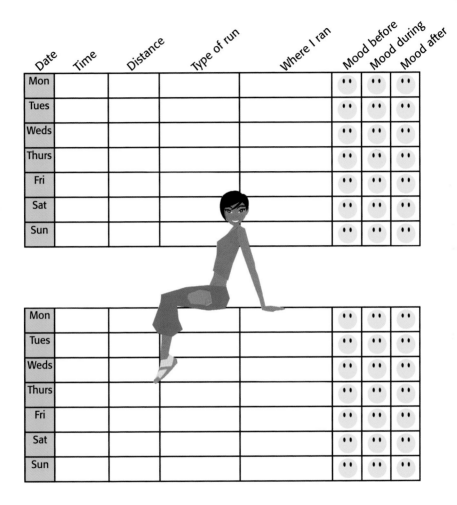

Date	Time	Distance	Type of run	Where I ran	Mood before	Mood during	Mood after
Mon					😊	😊	😊
Tues					😊	😊	😊
Weds					😊	😊	😊
Thurs					😊	😊	😊
Fri					😊	😊	😊
Sat					😊	😊	😊
Sun					😊	😊	😊

Date	Time	Distance	Type of run	Where I ran	Mood before	Mood during	Mood after
Mon					😊	😊	😊
Tues					😊	😊	😊
Weds					😊	😊	😊
Thurs					😊	😊	😊
Fri					😊	😊	😊
Sat					😊	😊	😊
Sun					😊	😊	😊

> 66 The only place where success comes before work is in the dictionary. 99
>
> Vidal Sassoon, legendary hairdresser

Date	Time	Distance	Type of run	Where I ran	Mood before	Mood during	Mood after
Mon							
Tues							
Weds							
Thurs							
Fri							
Sat							
Sun							

					Mood before	Mood during	Mood after
Mon							
Tues							
Weds							
Thurs							
Fri							
Sat							
Sun							

> 66 Running is like medicine – sometimes it tastes good, sometimes it doesn't, but it always makes you feel better afterwards. 99
>
> Gail Marcus, managing director

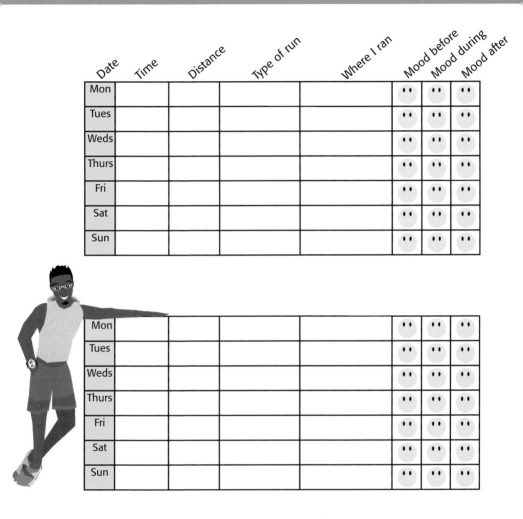

Date	Time	Distance	Type of run	Where I ran	Mood before	Mood during	Mood after
Mon							
Tues							
Weds							
Thurs							
Fri							
Sat							
Sun							

Date	Time	Distance	Type of run	Where I ran	Mood before	Mood during	Mood after
Mon							
Tues							
Weds							
Thurs							
Fri							
Sat							
Sun							

❝Remember, you can run and many cannot and will not run. Some people have never known what it's like to run. Make the most of it while you can.**❞**

Frank Horwill, international running coach

217

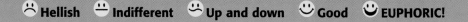

😖 **Hellish** 😐 **Indifferent** 😣 **Up and down** 😌 **Good** 😊 **EUPHORIC!**

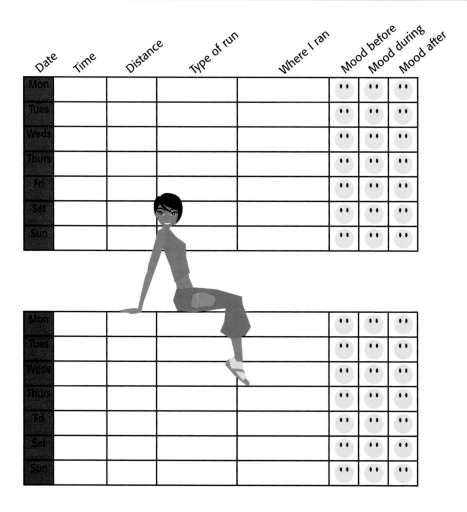

Date	Time	Distance	Type of run	Where I ran	Mood before	Mood during	Mood after
Mon							
Tues							
Weds							
Thurs							
Fri							
Sat							
Sun							

Date	Time	Distance	Type of run	Where I ran	Mood before	Mood during	Mood after
Mon							
Tues							
Weds							
Thurs							
Fri							
Sat							
Sun							

> **❝It's hard to beat a person who never gives up.❞**
>
> Babe Ruth, baseball legend

	Hellish		Indifferent		Up and down		Good		EUPHORIC!

Date	Time	Distance	Type of run	Where I ran	Mood before	Mood during	Mood after
Mon							
Tues							
Weds							
Thurs							
Fri							
Sat							
Sun							

Mon							
Tues							
Weds							
Thurs							
Fri							
Sat							
Sun							

66 The vision of a champion is someone who is bent over, drenched in sweat, at the point of exhaustion, when no one else is watching. 99

Anson Dorrance, women's football coach

☹ **Hellish**   😐 **Indifferent**   😕 **Up and down**   🙂 **Good**   😄 **EUPHORIC!**

Date	Time	Distance	Type of run	Where I ran	Mood before	Mood during	Mood after
Mon					😐	😐	😐
Tues					😐	😐	😐
Weds					😐	😐	😐
Thurs					😐	😐	😐
Fri					😐	😐	😐
Sat					😐	😐	😐
Sun					😐	😐	😐

Mon					😐	😐	😐
Tues					😐	😐	😐
Weds					😐	😐	😐
Thurs					😐	😐	😐
Fri					😐	😐	😐
Sat					😐	😐	😐
Sun					😐	😐	😐

> 66 Most look up and admire the stars.
> A champion climbs a mountain and
> grabs one. 99
>
> Henry Jackson Brown Jr, writer

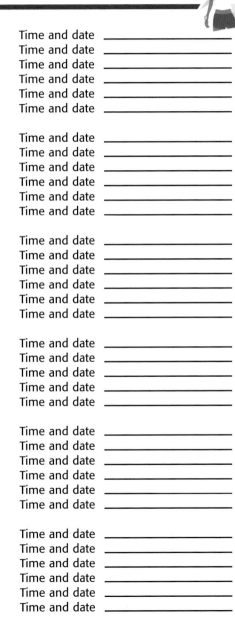

My personal best list

Knowing you're getting faster can be an incredible motivator. Record your personal best times (PBs) here to see how much you've improved.

Best time for 1.6km/1 mile

Time and date _____
Time and date _____
Time and date _____
Time and date _____
Time and date _____
Time and date _____

Best time for 5K/3 miles

Time and date _____
Time and date _____
Time and date _____
Time and date _____
Time and date _____
Time and date _____

Best time for 8km/5 miles

Time and date _____
Time and date _____
Time and date _____
Time and date _____
Time and date _____
Time and date _____

Best time for 10K/6 miles

Time and date _____
Time and date _____
Time and date _____
Time and date _____
Time and date _____

Best time for a half-marathon
(21km/13.1 miles)

Time and date _____
Time and date _____
Time and date _____
Time and date _____
Time and date _____
Time and date _____

Best time for a marathon
(42km/26.2 miles)

Time and date _____
Time and date _____
Time and date _____
Time and date _____
Time and date _____
Time and date _____

Contact us...

If this book has inspired you to take up running, or helped you get better at it, we'd really love to hear from you. Email us at lisa.jackson@natmags.co.uk or susie.whalley@natmags.co.uk and you may even be featured in a future edition of this book.

Read these...

- **Cross-Training For Dummies** by Martica Heaner and Tony Ryan, John Wiley & Sons, 2000
- **Eat Smart, Play Hard** by Liz Applegate, Rodale Books, 2001
- **Fitness On A Plate** by Anita Bean, A&C Black, 2003
- **Galloway's Book On Running** by Jeff Galloway, Shelter Publications, 2002
- **Lore Of Running** by Tim Noakes, Human Kinetics, 2003
- **No Need For Speed** by John Bingham, Rodale Books, 2002
- **Runner's World magazine** – to subscribe, call 01858 438844
- **The Complete Guide To Sports Nutrition** by Anita Bean, A&C Black, 2003
- **Zest magazine** – to subscribe, call 01858 438844

Visit these...

- www.runnersworld.co.uk
- www.serpentine.org.uk
- www.zest.co.uk

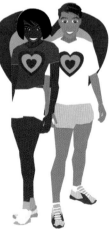

Run these...

- **Race For Life:** 0870 5134314, www.raceforlife.org
- **Run London Nike 10K:** www.runlondon.co.uk
- **BUPA races, such as the Great North Run:** www.greatrun.org or www.onrunning.com
- To apply for entry to the **Flora London Marathon**, pick up a free copy of *Marathon News*, a booklet available in sports shops such as JJB Sports and First Sport. For more entry info visit www.london-marathon.co.uk

A big thank you to...

▐▌▌▌➤ Rachel Boston, Abby Franklin, Marianne de Vries, Kelly Moseley and Kelly Flood for all their fantastic art and styling input.

▐▌▌▌➤ Thanks, too, to Miriam Hyslop, Helen Ponting and all at Anova Books, as well as Alison Pylkkänen, Emma Dally and all our wonderful colleagues at *Zest* and Natmags for their support and encouragement.

▐▌▌▌➤ This book looks as inspiring as it does due to the stunning still-life photographs of Louisa Parry and Derek Lomas and the wonderful illustrations of Paul Luke. Thanks, also, to Neil Cooper for shooting our fab cover.

▐▌▌▌➤ Thanks, too, to our eagle-eyed proofreader Libby Willis, for her untiring dedication to (and enthusiasm for) this book.

▐▌▌▌➤ Thanks to the experts who shared their expertise with us. Special thanks to Dr Dorian Dugmore (for further details of more advanced wellness testing, call 0161 9302477), Georgie Gladwyn at PhysioCentral, London, to Jon Roberts, Jane Wake, and Sammy Margo, to the experts who designed our running plans (Kirsty O'Neill, Joe Dunbar, Andy Ellis and Prof Tim Noakes), and to Prof Andrew Prentice for information about body-fat composition.

▐▌▌▌➤ Thanks, too, to all our wonderful case studies and the organisations that put us in touch with them: the Flora London Marathon (www.london-marathon.co.uk), Cancer Research UK (www.cancerresearchuk.org), Shelter (www.shelter.org.uk), Mind (www.mind.org.uk), Denis Tabakin at the Achilles Track Club (www.achillestrackclub.org), Slimming World (www.slimmingworld.com), Weight Watchers (www.weightwatchers.co.uk), Vittel (water sponsors of the Flora London Marathon), the American Cancer Society (www.cancer.org), Action On Addiction (www.aona.co.uk) and Victoria Brockhurst (www.thamesfitness.co.uk).

▐▌▌▌➤ And lastly, thanks to the hundreds of really enthusiastic runners from around the world who sent in contributions for this book and to the many people who bought the first edition of this book, used The 60-Second-Secret Plan to become runners and loved it so much that they turned many of their friends and family into runners, too!

Lisa and Susie

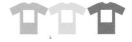

INDEX